Visit the Website: http://www.CancerA9YearStruggle.com

Reviews and Comments from Readers

"From the very beginning you are taken by the strong love that 2 people have for one another. When Tom and Irene were married, they vowed to each other that through good times and bad, sickness and health that they would always be there for one another. How so very true for this special couple. This book is a wonderful story for a caregiver or anyone faced with a family member or friend with a life threatening illness." --M.H.

"... I thought the book was wonderful and I believe there are a lot of lessons that can be learned from it, also, quite a bit of detailed information about cancer and the treatment of the disease... Your book actually gave me some insight into some of the things my Dad went through; for that, and for sharing your and Irene's story, I thank you." --R.B.

"Thank you so much for the book you wrote. It is truly a beautiful tribute to Irene and will be especially helpful for others that may be going through the same experiences." --G.&S.

"We finished reading 'Cancer: A 9 Year Struggle.' What a wonderful tribute to your life with Irene. The book was interesting reading and emotionally stirring. Thank you for sharing the journey with us." --T.&J.G.

"The new website is great Tom. I would just like to say, for those who haven't yet read it, that your book is a great guide for anyone who is facing a similar diagnosis and is afraid and not sure what to expect or how to handle it..." --B.E.

"... I really don't know what to say about Mr. Cooney's book. I really enjoyed reading a book about two normal people dealing with the daily ups and downs of one of life's greatest adversities. ...With that being said I feel that society as a whole would greatly benefit from Mr. Cooney's wonderful book being brought to life on the silver screen......" --S.R.

"The title may suggest otherwise but this is a story of life and love. The mechanics of a life with cancer are detailed, treatments, side effects, pain and the emotions attached to it all." --P.&K.S.

"I just read the book Tom. It is absolutely WONDERFUL! This book is truly the most beautiful true love story that I have ever read. Your writing style is perfect and the parts taken from Irene's journal entries make it very personal and heartfelt. I shed tears and I laughed too! Thank you again for sharing "your" Irene with all of us!" --C.K.

"Tom Cooney, Jr.'s book is a love story. Tom and Irene met at the Philadelphia Police Department. She was a student, he the instructor. They fell in love. Their journey has monumental challenges when Irene is diagnosed with colon cancer.... Tom and Irene will inspire anyone who ever had to make life changing decisions... It was easy to read... You will learn much about life and love. You will be better educated about the course of action to take should you or a loved one ever be diagnosed with this horrific disease." --L.F.

"Do you think "true love" or "soul mates" don't exist? Irene and Tom have a connection that transcends time. This book is truly the most beautiful true love story that I have ever read... A MUST-READ for everyone whether or not you share any experience with Cancer." --C.M.

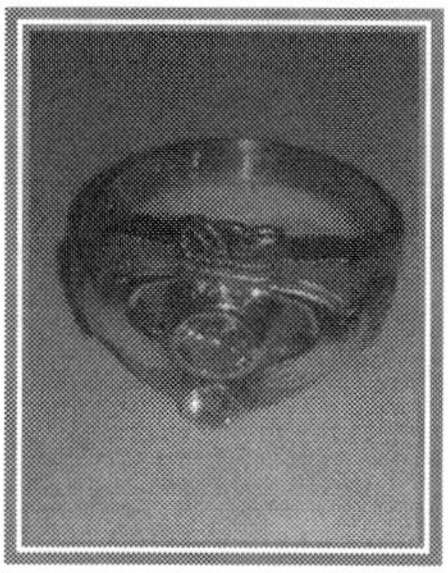

CANCER

A Nine-Year Struggle

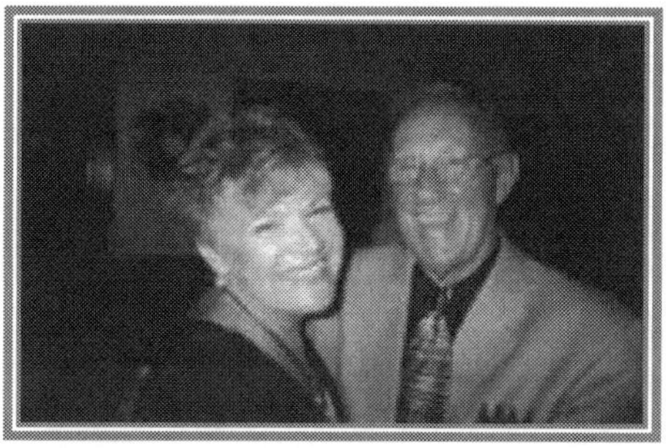

The Journey, after a Diagnosis of Fourth-Stage Cancer

As chronicled by a spouse, Tom Cooney Jr.

INFINITY PUBLISHING

ISBN 978-0-7414-8285-3 Paperback
ISBN 978-0-7414-8286-0 Hardcover
ISBN 978-0-7414-8287-7 eBook
Library of Congress Control Number: 2013901861

Printed in the United States of America

Published September 2013

INFINITY PUBLISHING
1094 New DeHaven Street, Suite 100
West Conshohocken, PA 19428-2713
Toll-free (877) BUY BOOK
Local Phone (610) 941-9999
Fax (610) 941-9959
Info@buybooksontheweb.com
www.buybooksontheweb.com

Contents

Dedicated to my wife,
Irene Cooney
January 31, 1953–June 22, 2012

Our Introduction

Irene struggled mightily for almost nine years, trying to get the most out of the rest of her life, once she was diagnosed with fourth-stage colon cancer in August 2003. She passed away June 22, 2012, after a very courageous and painful battle. I, as her husband, am delighted and happy she accepted her plight and refused to surrender to it. She remains as an inspiration to all our friends and family members whose lives she touched and who possibly may face illnesses of their own.

I chronicle our story and describe our many ups and downs as each phase of her treatment progressed through the years. I explain many of the side effects of her numerous chemo sessions, the major surgeries, and many other procedures. I depict some of Irene's responses to treatment in enough detail, including side effects, so people experiencing a diagnosis of cancer will be able to relate, especially when those side effects are too much for them to talk about or explain to family and friends.

We managed several trips during treatment, even twice to California wine country. We flew to Las Vegas and to Ireland. We made the best of any free time away from the hospitals and infusion rooms. We made deals with our medical team to delay a few days or skip a week of chemo so we could extend our mini-vacations. At times, we adjusted scheduled surgery to give us time through the holidays so we were home for Christmas. We carved out a few more days free of hospital stays and treatments whenever the opportunity arose.

Irene had periods in which there was "no radiological evidence of disease" or "no detectable hypermetabolic activity." In other words, the scans didn't show any cancer. Actually, it was lurking under the radar. We always took advantage of those breaks in treatment. Most of the time, however, we were terribly aware that Irene's disease was systemic and might reappear in the next PET or CAT scan.

Irene and I believed *quantity* would give us *quality*. People sometimes think they should focus the other way around. We didn't! We didn't have to make a decision between those two conditions, even though at times we were asked to confront it. But to us, *quantity* resulted in *quality*. We continued to hope for quantity. We tried to make our own quality.

My relationship with Irene started in 1999 during a seminar I was teaching. It was a prep course for police officers who wanted to score well on an upcoming detective's exam. I started a part-time business running those classes in 1984. I ran the business part-time until I retired from the Philadelphia Police Department in 1993. I then focused full time on developing and expanding the firm. I specialized in training, testing, and consulting for police and security organizations.

In that particular detective's prep course in 1999, I read the roll call, and a pretty, demure, woman answered to a specific surname. I thought how attractive she was and noticed that she wore a cute, sunny smile on her pretty face all the time. It wasn't a phony, plastic, politician's smile. A thought crossed my mind: *Maybe that's all it takes to be happy—wear a perennial happy face.*

I tried to do it myself, but it never worked for very long. It must come naturally. I discovered Irene always wore her soft smile in a natural way. She didn't have much in her life at that time to be very happy about, as I found out later, yet she always wore a pleasant smile.

During the seminar, Irene and I chitchatted now and then—teacher/student type conversations. But that was all. I thought about her, though—very pleasant thoughts. I was happy for her. Little did I know what was happening in her life. I knew almost nothing about her background, only her assignments and other requirements to register for my courses.

Well, the prep course ended after eight weeks, and then Irene was gone (but not forever), and she was not forgotten. I hoped she learned enough to be competitive on the exams, of course, but I missed her congeniality among the other students—and with me.

My background turned out to be very important in our relationship. I write the following words with both humility and a keen knowledge of my good fortune. During my years as an officer, I happened to be very successful in conquering the periodic promotional civil service exams administered by the city of Philadelphia. Later, this became very important during our struggle, because it gave me some stature for consulting and training in other smaller jurisdictions, thereby expanding my private business. And an important point: those elevations in rank also greatly increased my pension when I finally retired in 1993.

As the years zoomed by in the 1980s, long before I met Irene and while I was still wondering how I topped everyone else in the exams, I took advantage of opportunities that came my way. I designed and conducted promotional prep courses for various ranks of detectives, supervisors, and commanders. Eventually, as mentioned, I expanded my courses by topic and into other jurisdictions. That allowed me to retire from the police department in 1993 and coupled with my pension, I earned a comfortable living, devoting full time to teaching, consulting, and writing promotional prep manuals. This became crucial in the future, as it gave me the time and resources to be with Irene full time when she needed me the most.

Flavoring my relationship with Irene, once we became a couple, was my own fight with cancer. It added an important ingredient. In 1990, I was diagnosed with cancer. After two surgeries and a year of self-injections, I was back to normal—physically. One's worldview, however, changes after a cancer diagnosis. Being a cancer survivor gave me a personal understanding of the fear that the "Big C" diagnosis causes. That terrible moment never leaves you, when first you hear the doctor's words—from way down inside a dark, hollow tunnel, a voice gives you the bad news: cancer. The resultant fear shapes every thought for years to come.

It took a long ten years before my doctor finally told me I was in the clear. He still didn't use the word *remission*, though. I never heard that word from him; my doctor did not like to use the term. There is always a possibility that some of the cancer—a microscopic sliver of cells—is not totally removed during surgery and lingers there, waiting for some stimulant that enables it to begin reproducing and do new, more extensive damage.

You are never completely released, once the diagnosis is imposed on you. The fear always occupies your thoughts. Frequently, once diagnosed and cleared, people are stricken again. Similar thoughts continually floated through Irene's mind, never far from the surface. She feared most—and constantly worried throughout her ordeal—that the cancer might metastasize to her brain.

Irene's oncologists never used the word remission either. I never heard any oncologist use that word, except to say he didn't use the word, *remission*.

In writing this book, I obtained almost five thousand pages of documents and reports concerning Irene's treatments. The files include blood draws, surgeries (major and minor), diagnostic tests, and her astonishing number of chemo sessions. The pages and pages of reports also included information that doctors and nurses gathered from Irene's youth, which she had revealed in interviews. The doctors needed her entire medical history to establish baselines to determine a rate of progress—or lack of it—related to treatment regimens. They had to know every possible variable.

Delving into the records, I tried to count the number of infusions Irene endured over nearly nine years. The closest I could tally was approximately 175 *normal* chemotherapies. By "normal" I mean those cocktails commonly administered during treatment of cancer patients while in a cancer treatment center's infusion room. This number does *not* include take-home portable infusion pumps that dispense chemo cocktails over time, pills taken orally, or those infusions with new drugs or protocols in the Clinical Research Unit. Irene often experienced each of those types, but I didn't include those treatments in the total. She was infused through portable devices over many months in those years and participated in trials also.

Although the hospital records don't lend themselves to exact enumeration, I am certain that Irene's insurance companies have a precise number. (I didn't ask them for a summary.) My estimate is probably somewhat conservative, short of being totally accurate, but it doesn't matter for the purpose of this book. The significance is the sheer number of them and their horrid side effects.

I separated the pertinent pages of the hospital records into three big loose-leaf binders, one for each facility where Irene was treated. Then I broke them down further within the binders, by year of Irene's treatment. To prove a point again, in that several-inches-thick assortment of records from three different hospitals, I never read the word remission, even though Irene had several treatment breaks through the years, a couple of them lasting six months.

To us, "treatment break" was synonymous with remission. I mentioned earlier the common phraseology used, such as "no radiological evidence of disease." I think the word remission must have been invented in those TV series hospital dramas.

After my own experience with cancer in 1990, I focused for the following decade on my two sons and my business, thinking the rest of my life was going to be empty of a personal relationship—lonely, in other words. My two sons were still young, and they became the center of my universe from that moment on. Cancer changed my worldview.

Then, in early 2001, in an advanced detective prep course, there she was again. This time, she answered my roll call to a surname that was quite different ethnically from the name to which she answered in the first course.

Stasurak? I thought. *That wasn't her name back in '99. I wonder ...*

"Did you get married?" I asked her.

"No, sir, I got divorced."

That was the beginning of my life together with Irene. And ever since that moment in 2001, despite all we faced in the future, I wouldn't have changed places with anyone. I treasure the relationship I had with Irene—sweet, delightful, smiling Irene. Later, I loved reciting a particular Shakespearean sonnet to her and watching the love in her eyes. From a personal perspective, I went from fallow, emotional starvation to complete fulfillment.

In the pages following, I describe our nine-year journey. Irene, in a manner, is my coauthor. You'll notice many of her italicized "notations" throughout this book. Those comments are from a loosely kept journal we maintained. The entries bring Irene back into my life as I create this tribute to her. She is by my side as I sit at the computer, and she invites you to peek over my shoulder as I guide you through our nine year trek, with all its hills and valleys. I emphasize the amazing strength and endurance Irene summoned in order to withstand every torment cancer forces on the afflicted.

Finally, for those of you who have not confronted the disease personally, I pray that you and your loved ones are never threatened with it. For those readers who are beginning a fight against cancer, I hope you will find enough resolution, courage, and strength in this book to get more out of life, despite your illness. For the reader whose loved one battled and lost, I hope and pray you find some comfort and solace in these pages, for you are not alone.

Tom Cooney Jr.
Orlando, Florida

Postscript: Happy birthday and happy anniversary, Irene. I hope you like the book, honey.

Chapter One

Getting to Know Irene—and Me

"Break time!"

The seminar intensified during the first two hours. Most of the detective candidates needed to clear their minds of the investigative techniques they absorbed—or, in some cases, tried to absorb. The students headed to a couple of vending lunch trucks that usually parked outside the Philadelphia Police Academy classrooms, where I held classes. They were a handy, rolling cafeteria for attendees.

I got the approval of the deputy commissioner of the Training Bureau in the Philadelphia Police Department to use the classroom space, but there was a proviso: there had to be a sizable discount for the candidates competing in the departmental promotional exams. I happily extended reduced tuition to the Philly officers, supervisors and commanders, especially because of the free lease I was offered when I complied.

"Do you want anything from the lunch trucks, Inspector?" Irene approached my desk with a very nice smile. Her face seemed to glow.

"Yes, please, Irene—an egg salad sandwich and small chocolate milk."

I pulled out a few dollars. Irene refused to take my money; she smiled and said I should consider her generosity as the proverbial apple for the teacher. I really liked her. She returned in a few minutes and she, too, had an egg salad sandwich and chocolate milk.

We have something in common, I thought happily. *Egg salad sandwiches!*

We talked for the rest of the fifteen-minute break, I at my desk and she in the student seat in the front row.

In our chat over the sandwiches, I learned her divorce became final in late 1999—that was during the time she'd attended the first class. She added that she'd just purchased a small but quaint row home in a blue-collar neighborhood. She and her mother, Maria, who lived with her, were fixing it up. Her mother was seventy-six at the time. Born in the Ukraine, her mother had come to the United States in 1951 with her husband and three children. Irene, the fourth sibling, was born in America in 1953.

"Wow! That's very interesting," I said. "I would love to interview your mother. I'm sure she has a lot of great stories."

I meant the comment primarily as an expression of admiration toward Irene's mother. At the same time, I was intellectually curious. Think of it: Irene's mother had been born and then raised under the yoke of Communism, and on top of that, she'd lived through the German invasion of her native land. I didn't actually believe, however, such an interview was likely to happen. I was inquisitive, without any doubt, but although I wanted to invite myself to their home, I didn't do so. And then it happened.

Irene said, "Come on down!"

Without thinking I blurted out, red-faced, "Be glad to."

So I started visiting Irene and her mother in the quaint little row house on Lardner Street in Philadelphia. Irene learned being red-faced is a very common condition for me.

Today, I'm into my mid-seventies, and I'm still a blusher. I feel the blood going to my face, and my entire body heats up. I try to ignore it, but I blush at everything: praise, criticism, or meeting someone for the first time. I blush if I sense someone I'm talking to is having an uncomfortable moment—I blush for him or her. I'm not a liar, but if I were, detection would be instantaneous.

But I live with "the blush." Others may misinterpret my habitual response to both internal and external environmental stimuli. Those who believe a blush only indicates a lie must have thought every word coming out of my mouth was a non-truth. As time went by, Irene was touched by my blushing. I even blushed when she told me that! She said it endeared me to her even more. I suppose it was much the same as her ever-present soft smile endeared her to me.

Before long, all three of us—Irene, her mother, and I—were getting along nicely. I was a guest in their home. I was breaking bread with them—and taking notes. I was learning quite a bit about Irene through our combined conversations over some of the yummiest home-cooked meals I'd eaten in a long time.

I believe I can best introduce Irene to the reader by relating details about her mother and their relationship. You can gain a deeper insight by knowing her mother and the environmental influences in both their lives. I think you'll begin to love her mother, too, as I did over the years. After Irene and I married in 2005, Maria lived with us for years, until Irene became bedridden more often than not.

What an experience Irene's mother lived through! Born in the early 1920s, Maria was an infant when Stalin took over the reins in the USSR. She was ten and eleven years old in 1932–34 when an estimated six million to seven million Ukrainians starved to death. She knew many of them; they'd been her playmates. Maria vividly and scornfully remembered what the Soviet authorities called a famine. She saw the emaciated bodies in streets and streams, caused by her government in its futile utopian attempt at making everyone "equal." And of course, as George Orwell demonstrated in *Animal Farm*, there always were some who were more "equal" than others.

"The Communists told us everybody would be equal," Maria once explained. "True! We were all equally *poor* under that bureaucratic system. The party members did fine, though."

I loved listening. Irene also listened attentively.

Today, it is well authenticated that Stalin knew his policies were causing starvation among those pesky (in his mind) Ukrainians who were always trying to break away from Moscow's controlling influence. The Ukrainians wanted to gain their own independence.

On January 20, 1934, Maria saw her father (Irene's grandfather), Zacharko Skala, shot to death in his tiny kitchen for "hoarding" the swept-up bits of grain to make bread for his family. He'd hidden those little crumbs behind a cabinet. But those were "the people's" crumbs;

the tidbits were "for the people." A devoted party member in the village, the local delegate, told the regional party commissar about the "theft." Repercussion was swift and ruthless.

During the same period, Stalin purged an estimated ten thousand politically suspect officers from the military so he could install his minions in key ranks. Some of those killed were from Maria's village.

Maria explained that a failed agricultural program, a "cooperative" system, took the products of hard labor from the weary farmers and sold them to foreign nations to raise money for domestic programs. The government always tried to get bigger by giving out more and more "goodies" to certain people and party members for the benefit of the common good but at the expense of others.

"Goodies"? She described the Communist governmental programs as "goodies." This is great! I love this little woman.

Family farms became the "people's farms." Millions of farmers were not on the list to receive any wheat, corn, grain, or any other gains from the sale of those products to other nations. The proletariat, the "workers," along with the politicians and bureaucrats, were awarded the goodies. They built the military machine and tended the administration of the vastly growing government. Other groups, including Ukrainian farmers, were not included in the privileged classes. The major metropolitan population centers became the strongholds of "the party," not the expansive rural countryside and agricultural acreage in the Ukraine.

Maria Stasurak (nee Skala), Irene's mother, was nineteen when the Nazis blitzed most of the Ukraine with their tanks and artillery. They charged beyond Kiev, the closest large city to Maria's little farming village of Pomynyk. They were on their way to a failed attempt to capture the oil fields to the east to fuel their Panzers and Luftwaffe.

Irene's upbringing was rooted in those very scary days as Maria was trying to survive. Irene was a survivor, as she showed for almost nine years.

In 1942, at the age of nineteen, Maria was swept up by the Germans during their blitz and transported back to Deutschland to support the war effort in food production. Irene's mother spent the rest of World War II on a farm outside Riedensburg in the tiny hamlet of

Hattenhofen. She became one of the lost souls of the Third Reich's forced labor population, all from conquered lands.

A few weeks later, in 1942, after her long train and cart ride to Hattenhofen, another Ukrainian, Ivan Stasurak, was dumped onto that small farm. Maria and Ivan "married." The family always joked about that, despite her producing a certificate from a Catholic priest. It didn't stop the good-natured teasing, though. Their firstborn, a boy, opened his eyes on that little farm as a prisoner, like his mother and father.

The war ended in Europe in May 1945. The Red Cross and the occupying American forces took over the massive administration of several millions of the "displaced persons" (DPs) scattered throughout the geography previously controlled by the Nazi machine.

For six more years, the family was among the DP population staying in makeshift encampments in Germany. During that period, the second boy and a girl were born at two different farm sites. Those children first opened their eyes in the late 1940s, after the war was over.

In 1951, full of dreams, Maria, Ivan, and their three children sailed off to America on an American troop ship. They settled in Philadelphia. In 1953, Irene, the last of the Stasuraks' nuclear family, was born—the first to be born in the USA. When I later married Irene Stasurak, she became Irene Cooney.

Maria and Ivan's background had a strong influence on Irene's worldview. Even more, it developed Irene's strength, fortitude, and perseverance.

Adding to my enjoyment of spending time with Irene and her mother was my abundant interest in Eastern European culture. I minored in history at Temple University. To me, this entire story was fascinating. (I computerized data from the Stasurak family tree and later inserted the fuller ancestry into the Family Tree software program.)

At my very first visit, while Maria and I were talking, Irene made us dinner. It was the best steak I ever ate, marbled and juicy. She prepared it perfectly. After dinner, we three sat out on the rear deck of their tiny home and drank a few chilled glasses of wine as we looked out through the trees. Their rear view was a cemetery, a playground for neighborhood cats and the two toms belonging to Irene and her mother.

Maria drank her own homemade "medicine." I tried it. It was very, very tasty!

I'm actually having a date. And so are Irene and Maria. I like this setting. What a great evening.

I no longer had cancer, everyone I cared about was happy and healthy, and my two sons were both continuing their education. Tommy was twenty-three and Chris was eighteen at the time. I'd been divorced from my sons' mother since 1984. She and I were getting along just fine. Life was good.

After many visits to Irene's, I almost—but not quite—asked Irene to go to Florida with me to attend a niece's wedding. It included a five-hour cruise on a casino pleasure ship. I was too shy to ask, though, and I thought it was too forward of me at the time. For years afterward, Irene lightly scolded me for not asking her then for a first "real date." She'd wink at me, implying our romance would have ignited earlier.

I reflected for the first time in years that my personal future might be looking up. The empty feeling was slowly dissipating. Emotionally, I started feeling more uplifted. It was a nice feeling—one I hadn't had for as long as I could remember. Irene was so comfortable to be around in every way. My clenched jaws were relaxing for the first time in years.

There was no sparring between us to gain control or dominate. We did not compete with each other in any way. Neither of us was interested in who was boss, who was right, or who would win an argument. There were no arguments! It wasn't important. Neither of us tried to change the other. I had "man" things to do, and Irene had "woman" things she liked to do. We were content in our old-fashioned, old-world, traditional ways. It was easy. It was not combative at all. Neither of us was looking to "find" ourselves. That search was long over. For me, it was effortless and calm to be around her. It remained that way to the very end, even throughout the entire period of her illness.

Irene, her mother, and I had dates similar to that first one many more times during 2001 and 2002. I couldn't bring myself to believe Irene and I were an "item" just yet, and I acted accordingly. I did not push myself on Irene.

Later, I told her how interested I was early on but that I had no hope she would consider me as a partner in a serious relationship. For one thing, I was fifteen years older. I was enjoying her companionship only. Subsequently, she too admitted her interest but had no hope for a deeper relationship. She believed I probably dated assistant DAs and professional women only—she was "just" a cop. That was very far from the truth.

I was born and raised in a blue-collar neighborhood. At one low point, 1947–48, I lived in a project for a year and a half. I had no pretensions about my roots or status. A policewoman would be fine with me. Irene didn't know that, and I didn't tell her so. We were still not an item yet.

Then, suddenly, in August 2002, I got a surprising phone call from Irene. She placed high on the detectives' promotional list, and she wanted to thank me for the help she'd received through the classes. One other startling comment she added:

"I'm retiring and moving to Florida to be closer to my sister and brothers. My mother wants to be near them, too. She's getting older and misses them."

I knew Irene's father had passed away in 1985, and Irene would do anything for her mother—even uproot herself, if that's what her mother needed. She was dedicated to Maria, who stretched to reach five feet tall but ate voraciously. Maybe Maria's appetite was stimulated by memories of much leaner days. Maria was as unique as Irene was. I cared for them both by this time, but I understood why a move to Florida would interest them. But why so suddenly?

"There are a lot of things going 'round in my head," she explained. "I need to get away too."

In her personal life, maybe? I wondered. *I won't ask.*

"Maybe we can have *cawfee* before I leave, Tom," she suggested.

I loved that Philadelphia accent. Coffee was "cawfee"; water was "wawder." I like accents of any flavor.

"Definitely," I responded. "But you placed so high on the detective's exam." I still wasn't being forward with my feelings. I was awkward around her, even over the phone. "Well, you know that I have a place outside Orlando, Irene. Where are you moving?"

"Bradenton. It's over on the west coast near Tampa. My sister, her husband, and my nephew bought a house nearby their houses. They're going to rent it to me. There's just a little fixing up to do. We'll have something in common, Tom. We'll both be Floridians."

"Yes. But you just finished fixing up your home on Lardner Street. You sure are a worker bee. Bradenton—that's about two hours away from my place. Can I ride over to see you when I'm down there?"

"I was *hoping* you would suggest that, Tom."

Am I hearing things? I wondered. And then I asked, "When are you leaving?"

"In a few days."

I was trying to think of when I was returning to my home in Florida so I had an excuse to drive to Bradenton. "Well, Irene, I'll make sure I visit you soon. I'm already planning to go back down south for about a week."

"Good. I'll be looking forward to seeing you."

Irene laughed a little. I could sense her smile and pleasant face even over the phone. She said she would e-mail me her address. We hung up.

Rewind a few years, so I can explain my situation at that moment when I got that call from Irene. I bought the home near Orlando late in 1996 and settled it in January 1997. I intended to retire and actually did retire in my mind. I was more or less just wrapping it up in Philly. I actually established residency in Florida in 1997 and was commuting to Philadelphia regularly to conduct my seminars. I wrote consultation reports from my home office in Florida and communicated, if need be, using the Internet and phone, with an occasional flight to Philly.

I put my home in Somerton Springs, Philadelphia, up for sale. It took more than a year to sell it. The market was rather slow. When it did sell in late 1998, the only home I owned was in Florida. I retired for a while until I started another business.

I formed a sole proprietorship, bought several virtual-reality golf machines, and over time, placed them in various locations around the Orlando area. The locations were ill suited, however, and patrons caused a lot of recurring damage. I should have placed them in country clubs, where they might have been better appreciated. Nevertheless, eventually I rid myself of all but one of them. I keep that one in the garage to remind me of the fiasco that adventure turned out to be. It's still in the garage.

I was eventually drawn back to Philly to fulfill a couple of contracts that were too good to refuse. I decided to rent an apartment in order to establish an office and living space up north. That's where I was when I received that life-changing phone call from Irene in August 2002, when she told me she was retiring and heading south.

Fast-forward this time to the following day after that particular phone call.

Late that afternoon, I got a second phone call. This time it was from Irene's close friend—I knew her as well. Sandy was in an academy class sometime in the early '80s when I was assigned there as an instructor. Sandy kept in touch not only with me but also with everyone else she ever met in her life, it seemed to me. She retired from the police department and took a job in security in an Atlantic City casino.

Irene was with Sandy during that fortuitous second phone call, the day before Irene was to leave for Florida. They asked me to take a ride down to the casinos and have dinner with them. One of their friends, an Atlantic City cop, was celebrating a birthday. It was as good an excuse as any for me to be with Irene before she and her mother departed, and it was only an hour away, so I jumped at it.

Sandy got us into some exclusive areas within the casinos on the strength of her security badge. That was interesting.

I am forever grateful to Sandy for her role in bringing Irene and me together that beautiful evening in the Irish Pub in the heart of Atlantic City. We dined with the friends from the Atlantic City PD. Then, wonderfully and fatefully, Irene came home to Philadelphia with me. We finally became an item. We were both finally ready, as they say, after many months of our quiet dates on Lardner Street. I began to think,

Are the pieces of my life finally fitting together? Neither one of us may ever face loneliness again. There may be an exciting new world out there for us. I'm beginning to feel good about this—I think.

The very next day, I was helping her move—very exciting and depressing at the same time!

As an aside, when Irene retired and sold the cute little row house with a cemetery view in the rear, she had a very nice assignment in the District Attorney's Office in the Insurance Fraud Unit—mostly day work and soft clothes. She was leaving a very enviable position. Irene had the alias of "Kathy Falcone." Once, while sitting in a doctor's office—the doctor was under investigation—and thinking and musing over her life's experiences, she forgot her alias. It took a couple times of the receptionist's repeating, "Ms. Falcone," before it dawned on Irene that *she* was Ms. Falcone. I imagined and hoped when I heard the story that she'd been daydreaming pleasant thoughts while that permanent smile was forming on her lips. The fraud investigation was successful, nevertheless, in spite of Irene's momentary lapse.

Back in 1990, when Irene graduated from the police academy, she was assigned to the 25th District and then later to the 7th District. Irene first met Sandy in the 7th District. Irene met up with her again in the Insurance Fraud Unit.

Sandy helped Irene and her mother move out of Irene's home when Irene separated from her first husband. Irene and Maria just picked up and left, wondering where they were going to stay. No worries! They stayed with Sandy for a while. A few years later, in 2006, after Irene and I moved permanently to Florida, we also stayed with Sandy in her Atlantic City condo on one of our trips up north. She was a very frequent caller during the entire period Irene was ill.

Irene's separation/divorce period was 1999–2000. Irene and Maria moved from small apartment to small apartment until she bought the cute little house on Lardner Street. Mother and daughter settled down, happy to have a floor beneath them, a roof overhead, and a bedroom for each of them.

Sandy told me of that unsettled period in their lives. I pictured two women on a dirty, snow-covered city street at sundown; one older, one younger; carrying suitcases and leaning into the wind. I imagined the pair covering and protecting their eyes from blasts of mixed snow and sleet that whirled around. Both wore a determined expression on their faces, but they were smiling, even though their destiny was unknown to them. I saw them bravely confronting whatever came around the next wind-blasted corner.

In fact, earlier in their lives, during Irene's first marriage, her mother and Irene cleaned houses to make a dollar. Nothing was beneath this pair of hardy Ukrainian ladies in the effort to put food on the table. Both were proud women. No wonder the Germans lost the war on the Eastern Front.

Irene and her sister, Tammy, opened a hair salon before Irene became a police officer. They worked very long hours in order to make ends meet. After Irene divorced, always smiling, she still cut hair part-time in the basement of the little home on Lardner Street. On the day I was helping Irene move south, I relaxed and took a breather in the barber chair.

Irene came to the Advanced Detective Course in 2001. That's when she invited me to interview her mother and have dinner at her newly purchased row home. That's when our lives intertwined for the rest of her days.

Saddened and a little confused, I helped load Irene's car and then watched as she drove off with her mother and her cats. The very packed car pulled out of the rear driveway that separated the cemetery from the block-long row of cozy homes, and they began the 1,150-mile journey to their new lives. They were bravely facing the unknown again.

I stood there for a while. I thought maybe there was a new chance for me too—I hoped. I missed her already. I was so glad I'd bought the house near Orlando, just a couple hours from Bradenton. Standing there in the rear driveway, I dreamed of when I would see Irene again.

I conjured up a thought or two about all those long-deceased people lying under the weather-beaten grave markers. *I wonder! Are there hopeful messages rising from that sacred acreage? Are any of those souls trying to cross over?*

Squirrels zipped around and frantically tried to find their acorns and discover new spots to later bury them. The squirrels and Irene would survive, though, for a while longer.

I'll see you again soon, Irene. I hope.

I didn't know then what I know now. In August 2003, a year or so after they moved, Irene and Maria dealt with something far more dreadful than dusk on a lonely winter city street—as would I.

My Quirks

Now you know a bit about Irene. I think it is very important for you to understand what motivated her to endure so much in her life and throughout her illness. Irene's deep caring for her mother and Maria's love for Irene were important factors in my overall impression of Irene.

Another reason I was fascinated with this daughter and mother team: her Eastern European heritage intrigued me.

Soon after I graduated from high school, I joined the US Air Force to see the world. At the time, in the mid-1950s, the Soviet Union was the enemy. The Cold War was heating up quite a bit. In the service, I received training in two specialties: electronic countermeasures (ECM) and radio traffic analysis (RTA). I was schooled in Russian/Soviet geography, history, politics, major population centers, and of course, their military and all that entailed. I spent time in Europe and in Turkey, among other places. You can probably guess what my primary responsibilities were.

I started night school in 1960 at Temple University (BA '72), after I was honorably discharged from active duty. And I became so interested in continuing to study that particular culture that I started reading several of the Russian writers. The nineteenth-century authors were high on my list, as were the twentieth-century ex-patriots and exiles. I always had time for Shakespeare too.

Naturally, I was steeped in my own Irish roots. *The Story of the Irish Race* by Seumas MacManus—massive at more than seven hundred pages—was a definitive work. I had a keen interest in my own ethnicity.

Saturated with that background, I developed a personal theory: Eastern European and Irish would make good friends and mates with each other. Irish and Ukrainian history shared similar tragedy and oppression for hundreds of years. The Irish always were striving for independence. So were the Ukrainians and most of the other twentieth-century satellite nations within Eastern Europe. Individual liberty is in the DNA and soul of both peoples. Both cultures have, to this day, a huge capacity for suffering, often defined in much of their literature. When you finish reading this book, you'll understand Irene suffered greatly and handled it all with grace until the day she died.

Additionally, I was assigned for a few years in the 1970s to the Homicide Division when I was a detective. That specialty requires a heavy need for interview and interrogation skills. To make it easier to size up a subject, I came up with a Psych 101 cookie-cutter approach. It's a simplistic template, but I found it often worked in quickly getting the most information from either witnesses or suspects. It still works for me in my everyday life, too. It also was important when I was initially sizing up Irene, through force of habit. After a short time, I threw out the template in Irene's case. I didn't need it any more. I was, indeed, falling in love. There's no cookie-cutter shortcut available in the world of romance.

Now give me a few minutes to inform you about my quirks. I don't believe they are considered mainstream in this neo-modern day and age of conformity.

If I were king and a dictator, the phrase "I'm offended" would be one I would eliminate from the language—or used only in really, really extraordinary situations. I can't think of a circumstance in which *I* would use it. As a police officer, I've experienced some nasty, intended insults, but I was never offended. I think people who use that phrase are less well adjusted than they would have us believe. They need to get over being a victim.

"That's not fair" would be another retort I would ban, if I were a tyrant. My parents ensured I stopped using the phrase by the time I was in first grade. It's slightly annoying for me to hear parents insisting their spoiled child isn't being treated fairly. Even Dr. Spock refuted his own theories regarding self-esteem before he died. Irene told me she felt the same way. I knew she meant it. What a relief!

I think you should have some idea of the world I come from, which may explain why I was alone for a while until I met Irene. As my sons were growing up, each one, at some point, said, "Dad, I'm bored." Well, that didn't sit well with me. I simply responded, "That's your fault." I told them I didn't want to hear them say that to me again. I continued, in a calm tone, so each understood what I meant. It is up to him, not others, to keep himself entertained or busy. I added, "Don't lay guilt trips on anyone, including me!"

I never heard my boys use those words again—around me. They don't blame others for anything either. They accept responsibility, unlike many politicians. Good leaders don't blame others. In fact, my sons complain about being *too* busy. Excellent! My fatherly advice worked. You can assume if you mention the phrase "I'm bored" around me, I form an opinion about you, and it's probably that you are spoiled—unless you immediately take the bull by the horns *yourself* and don't require anyone else to entertain or cater to you.

Irene never told me or anyone else in my earshot that she was bored, treated unfairly, or offended. Not from the very first day I met her, long before she had any idea of my quirks. Not up to the last day of her life. It's bad, bad news for a man to become entangled with a self-centered woman, and vice versa.

I never warned her not to use the "bored" word around me. She was never bored with the kind of life she was leading. She was taking care of her mother, and that gave Irene strength. She had someone to love and to work hard for. You're never bored when you love someone deeply and unconditionally—that's a fact! You're always thinking of the other person. You're not usually thinking about yourself except for basic, normal necessities. But it requires being *able* to love someone more than yourself. It's too bad that particular capability is so rare. Most parents have it for their children, of course, but unfortunately, maybe not for their spouses.

Enough about what makes me tick. What follows is far more important.

Gateway to Her Personality: Irene's Smile

Irene sported a permanent smile. It was attractive. It attracted me. In addition, when I initially sized up Irene (I don't ask people what their Zodiac sign is), I found she possessed loads of common sense. I wasn't walking on eggshells or dancing around any controversial issues. It was no effort at all to be around her. No continual sparring existed as to who was right or wrong. And neither one of us was the least bit star-struck regarding famous personalities. That was important to me. Irene had grown well beyond that teeny-bopper phase. It's a pity so many adults have not. Both of us were old school in our beliefs, values, and customs.

While I admire *assertive* women, *aggressive* women are annoying and too egocentric for me. What's the difference? An aggressive woman intrudes; an assertive woman does not. An aggressive woman tells her escort she can open that door herself without his help. Irene would say, "Thank you," in response to the courtesy. Irene didn't feel threatened by such gestures. She appreciated them. I'm so sorry I got out of the habit of opening doors for Irene. I shouldn't have allowed that to happen. But Irene didn't complain.

An assertive woman says, "I want to open a hair salon." On top of that, she would say, "I want to become a police officer, then a detective, and eventually a captain." She then would step *quietly* onto the path that gets her where she wants to go. No one needs to get out of her way. She doesn't feel compelled to ensure that everyone understands where she is coming from.

The assertive woman knows what she wants and does something about it. She doesn't intrude and police the speech, eating habits, or shoe color of others. She doesn't worry about how much money someone else has in her pocket; she only worries about how much is in her own. She doesn't even let cancer stop her if she wants to paint the house or get a job at Home Depot. (You'll soon see!)

By the way, Irene did not object at all when I called her "honey" and "sugar." Call Irene Miss, Ms., or Mrs.—she was just fine with any of those, although she preferred Mrs. after we were married. That made me relax. I didn't have to be careful what I said around her.

Another very important personality trait that Irene possessed was independence. Irene was not defiantly independent; that's aggressive, immature, and the kind of independence teenagers believe brings freedom. She liked being a little different from the crowd. In her mature years, she felt no compulsion to follow the latest trends. She could say either yes or no. She was secure and independent in a subtle way, yet assertive if necessary. Many incidents proved it to me.

She was very comfortable in her own shoes. She didn't think she knew everything. She didn't feel superior to anyone, consciously or unconsciously. She had an open mind but remained able to sort things out for herself. She was easygoing. Everyone felt comfortable around her.

She loved deeply when she loved. I know that for a fact. Irene was feisty when necessary. She once told someone, in a very loud and threatening tone, "Don't you *dare* talk to my husband that way!" She meant it. The individual who heard that command was very nice to me thereafter.

One other story: A juvenile going to and from school repeatedly walked across the golf course and then between our home and the house next door. It was a shortcut. It soon wore a path between the houses, and there was concern as well that he might get hit with a golf ball.

After we told him several times to walk the normal path along the sidewalk, he knocked over some stone borders on our property when we were not at home (we probably were at the hospital). Finally, out a window, we saw him performing his little trick and walking away. I got the camera and started videotaping him as he continued on his way.

Assertively, Irene said to me, "Let's go!" We kicked into cop mode, I guess. The kid started running. We jumped into the car and went after him. We stayed on the streets, naturally, while he cut across the golf course.

We caught up to him as he was about to go into his gated subdivision. I continued to film as we had a heated conversation. He knew I was still filming. Irene, in that assertive tone I'm sure she used while on duty (but only if necessary to control a situation), warned him of the law and statute he was breaking and the evidence we had—the video—loudly telling him that his future could be seriously damaged with an arrest.

She had a determined look on her face, but I swear I still saw that smile. Maybe the kid saw it, too, but she was very assertive.

When he retreated into his subdivision, an aggressive person would have screamed derogatory names to intimidate or insult him. Irene was always ladylike, without being a pushover, even when arresting someone, I'm told. She never swore. I liked that.

The next day, he knocked on our door and said he wanted me to videotape him as he replaced the stones he'd overturned. I started filming, and he apologized. He has never taken the shortcut again. Maybe he or a neighbor told his parents about the episode, and he was strongly advised to correct his ways. But Irene was certainly and obviously effective, too.

Irene vowed that when she and her mother went out on their own, no one would ever take advantage of her again. Those days are distant in her past. She gained even more confidence through her years on the police force. She never sat back and tolerated abuse in any way, nor did she allow anyone to abuse her man—me. Not that I couldn't handle any situation myself. Irene didn't often have to defend me. She liked it when I stood on my own two feet. I could always see her smiling.

We didn't find fault in each other either. She was proud of me, and I was proud of her. That seems to be unique among couples. At least, spousal pride is not expressed as often as it should be. It's wonderful if you can feel proud of your wife or husband. That special feeling is often a choice you consciously make, one way or the other. Love helps make that choice.

In normal situations, among family and friends, Irene was shy and modest but not quite a shrinking violet. When necessary, she had a very strong streak. I loved it!

The power or grace it takes for an individual to display the appropriate characteristic at the appropriate time in the appropriate circumstance takes years to learn—or it is truly a gift. And it came naturally to Irene. That is why everyone she met loved her, including me. She was remarkable in every way.

Irene was natural even down to her Philadelphia twang. Later, I would tell everyone the reason I married her was that I loved her "foreign" accent. I too have the same twang. I miss hearing Irene say, "Let's getta cuppa cawfee." I miss it terribly.

Be at ease if you think Irene spotted security with me and roped me in. It was natural for Irene and her mother to want stability and safety—who doesn't? And what man doesn't want to provide comfort for those he loves and then feel good about it? I've had enough relationships to be able to keep my wits about me in those situations. My life's experiences gave me useful insight into such circumstances.

To be sure of someone's affection, however, put it to the friends-and-family test. Irene and her mother both passed with flying colors. No one—not my sons, who are eagle-eyed and protective of their mother and me; not my sister and her family; not my brother and his wife and children; not anyone else in my extended family and circle of friends—doubted Irene's feelings for me. All, without exception, gave their blessing to our romance. Irene and her mother were keepers.

But here was the real clincher and a tip to every reader, male or female: the matter of snoring or having a night cough! Everyone probably snores now and then or even does so chronically. I know I do on occasion. I take a medication that causes a dry nighttime cough at times, too.

I've watched very irritating TV advertisements hawking snore and cough suppressors. The wife in the commercials is obviously annoyed, tossing and turning and sending body language signals to the intrusive partner, as if he can control the spasms. That doesn't happen until he discovers this new product that will save their marriage. She covers herself with her pillow and tosses and turns, letting her husband know just how upset she is. In one commercial, the man is forced to leave the room and settle on the sofa.

Well, Irene never, ever vocalized any frustration or sent any body language signals regarding my snoring or coughing. And she never implied that I should go to another room because she couldn't sleep. That is the ultimate test of caring and love. And let me add, I would love to hear *her* sweet, soft snores and her "talking in tongues" once again. But I hear nothing—nothing at all coming from her place in bed beside me. It is silent. There is only a noiseless silk rose on her pillow next to me. Think of that the next time you feel inconvenienced by noises coming from the person on the other side of your bed. Personally, I don't like the current silence.

In our relationship during this earlier period, there was something else that relaxed me when Irene and I talked about our pasts. When I was diagnosed with cancer in 1990, my children were very young. Tommy was thirteen and Chris was about eight and a half. I was concerned about my own survival and the welfare of my sons, in the event I didn't win my battle with the disease. I created a living trust in which I spelled out what I wanted to happen with any estate I had accumulated at the time I might meet my end. My children would split it 50/50 over time.

Irene fully understood that and actually said that was the way it should be. When we started living together, we split everything down the middle. Later, when we bought a house together, both our names were on the deed. She did not lean on me financially at all. She had a good income of her own at the time. We shared the mortgage and maintenance costs. We built equity, and when we sold the house three years later, we shared the proceeds.

If I had passed away first, those proceeds would have belonged to her, 100 percent, because they went into a joint account. She was happy and content with that arrangement. She had no designs on any assets I had acquired *before* we were a couple. I told her the way it was very early in our relationship. She did not bat an eye. Irene wanted it that way. She felt responsible for the future well-being of my children as if they were her own. Irene was the farthest thing from being a gold-digger. She was as generous in her own right as any person I ever knew.

Later, when we married in 2005 and after Irene was diagnosed with cancer a little less than two years earlier, I added her as a beneficiary to my insurance policies, my IRA, social security, and any other monetary assets I had. She then shared a three-way split with my sons.

If I was run over by a train, Irene would be taken care of, physically and financially. It was an important discussion. Now, once declared, that was a worry we put behind us.

Being a caregiver for Irene during her struggle with cancer was effortless for me; it was a privilege. I wanted to do it. I am hoping that if necessary, you will want to do it for your loved one and that you also will find it effortless. Maybe the situation will develop with your parents, a spouse, or another person you love.

During one of Irene's first visits to my home in Orlando, we sat on the lanai drinking coffee watching the sunrise. Listen in.

"Honey, you'd have made a great mother. My boys really enjoy you. You're so easy to be around and to love."

"Thank you, Tom. Your sons and I will always be close. I think highly of them. Who wouldn't? They're both very good boys—I mean, men. They were raised right."

Irene pointed at the brilliant rising sun that was casting long shadows of the oak trees across the pond behind the house. All the wild birds were coming to life and starting their day of feasting. An osprey made a swift dive into the pond, grabbed a fish and flew off into the sun.

"Wow! Look at that, honey. That bird will feed its family today. That's a great sunrise, isn't it?"

"I love this early morning view from the lanai, Tom. Thank you."

"Honey, you thank me for everything. You don't have to do that."

Irene always showed gratitude whether or not it was needed.

"I want to, Tom. I am so happy."

Chapter Two

The Return Trip from Florida

Six long months passed since Irene and her mother headed south. We grabbed many romantic opportunities to be together, both at her home in Bradenton and my home near Orlando. We celebrated a belated fiftieth birthday for Irene, and my neighbors got to know my love more than just in passing. They fell in love with Irene, too.

For my birthday gift to her, I had a star named for Irene through the International Star Registry. It's recorded in Switzerland and in the U.S. Copyright Office. Two large framed documents hang on the wall in our bedroom, attesting there is a bright and shining star named "Irene." One of them illustrates the coordinates and the star's position in the universe. The other is an ornate Certificate of Registry. We gazed into the clear heavens and admired the star every night. I still do.

I had settled the purchase of my Florida home in January 1997, mainly to escape the recurring brutal ice and snowstorms that Philly was bracing against. It was an ideal time for an investment, and my sister and her family just bought a nice home there to boot. I liked central Florida better than either coast. The Orlando suburbs gave easy access to the ocean or the Gulf for quick trips if we wanted to dip our toes, without putting up with the year-round congestion Disney World brings to the area.

The modern airport and Florida turnpike were convenient for my sons and other relatives when they took Florida vacations and stayed at my home. The younger members of my extended family always wanted to go to Uncle Tommy's to see Mickey and Minnie. A bonus for me was my house was on a new golf course. Several neighbors and I golfed regularly through those early years.

My sons and I were "Disneyed-out" after a few hectic years of park visits with our annual passes and subsequent free entries, courtesy of Disney cast members, my sister and brother-in-law. But we still loved our Florida vacation home for other reasons.

On occasion, before we were married, Irene and I drove leisurely back and forth between Florida and Philly, stopping along the way at interesting cities like Myrtle Beach and Charleston. We also dined on big grouper sandwiches down by the river in Savannah—very tasty!

Irene loved the home, too. Plenty of big, quarrelsome sandhill cranes paraded across the back of the property. Momma duck and her dozen or so ducklings waddled within five feet of the pool screen. A bald eagle lived in the conservation area and occasionally swooped down to grab a fish dinner from the pond behind the house to feed his family. Storks, cormorants, and other wildlife constantly kept us company.

We skinny-dipped in our pool on warm nights and during the hot days when no neighbors were around, which we hoped was often. On either side of our home, the families were "snowbirds"—some recently retired but still had beloved children and grandchildren up north they couldn't leave for more than a couple months at a time.

Our big lanai and pool with adjoining spa afforded relative privacy, given the configuration of the parcel—a pie shape with the broadest leg across the back, where we overlooked the large pond onto the seventeenth green. Our view then followed the eighteenth fairway, a long par 5. Our resident alligator's interaction with golfers always was amusing, too. He often sunned on the far bank of the pond behind the house, and when a golfer looking for a lost ball inadvertently approached him, both quickly would hustle away from each other in opposite directions. Farther over to the right was conservation land that was not developed.

It was very romantic in the evening, with the pool lighting and inside, by the fireplace in the family room, where we had the view through sliding glass doors. It does get cold in Florida during the winter for short periods. We loved dining along International Drive in Orlando, where there are some great steak houses—Charley's, for example.

My Florida golfing buddies and their families all told me that Irene was a keeper. When I was single, they were sometimes on the lookout to match me up. Once I met Irene, their search was over, as far as they were concerned. Our little group was close-knit for many years and consisted of the buyers of the first eight lots.

All of us bought at about the same time, as the homes were being built in 1996–97. We all moved in at that time, so it was easy to have impromptu parties around the holidays. Later, when Irene was a regular at the house, she would impress the gang with her hostess and culinary skills. Her king crab legs, lobster tails, and crab cakes were the best. Everyone who met Irene loved her—and her cooking!

Irene started cleaning up the Florida home when we met there and had spare moments. After all, my sons and I had lived and vacationed there. I didn't concern myself at all as to whether my sons would get along with Irene. It was automatic.

As time went by and we married, Tommy and Chris did not like to use the term stepmother. They called her Irene, of course, but referred to her as their mother-in-love. Irene lit up when she heard them say that, but she always hastened to tell them they had only one mother and one father. Then she would point to me. All was well in the land of Irene and Tom.

But when a few lucrative contracts came up that enticed me enough to rent a duplex from a friend in Philadelphia while I serviced the contracted agencies, I did it. I bought a bed and other miscellaneous furniture, including a small antique desk, which I eventually brought to Florida.

One of those contracts was issued by the Public Safety Department of a university in the area, which wanted to make some promotions in its growing police department. The school hired me to design, construct, and administer the entire exam process. The person in charge knew of my experience in that area. Later, Irene and my sons, as monitors, usually helped during the administering of the exams.

I sold my Philly house in Somerton Springs in late 1998. I'd owned it for twenty-one years. During my divorce in 1984, I borrowed the money to pay half its value to my former wife. I kept the house and moved my elderly parents in with me to get them out of a dangerous neighborhood. My ex-wife bought a nice single just four miles away. That was great for the children.

My father passed away a year later in 1985, at almost eighty years old. My mother lived on for ten years, treating my sons to her delicious meals and caring for me when I was recuperating from my cancer surgery in 1990. She was eighty-two when she died in 1995.

My parents' last years were a lot more comfortable than they'd ever known in their past. They were married in 1933, during the Great Depression, and started their family during that dire period. I wished they'd lived long enough to meet Irene. They would have instantly told me she was a keeper. Then again, maybe they have met her already.

Six months after Irene and Maria moved to Florida, I was in my office in the Philly duplex when I called Irene and asked her to come back up north with me, permanently, at least until both of us retired—again. She missed the camaraderie that a career in law enforcement provided, and she missed me. I loved that. She also needed the money and the economic security a law enforcement career would bring into her and her aging mother's life. Timing was perfect to seal the deal for her return. Irene returned to Philly in February 2003 to my two-bedroom duplex. Her mother came a few months later, when we bought a house in the Fox Chase section of Philadelphia.

The Philadelphia Police Department has a policy that a retired officer can return to service within a year after leaving, as long as the employee's last commanding officer approves the reinstatement. It gives the department first choice in selecting seasoned officers in preference over recruits in order to fill vacancies.

When Irene moved to Florida, she anticipated being hired by the Manatee County (Florida) Sheriff's Department or some other police agency in Florida. That did not work out as expected. Hiring in law enforcement in that area was a very slow process, and she had rent to pay. She made ends meet working at an Olive Garden Restaurant, serving tables, as the process dragged on. The move was a fizzle, financially, for Irene, and the future was not looking bright.

Irene spent a lot of money on a down payment and on furniture for that row home, plus the fixing-up expenses. In addition to the car in which she headed south that was packed full, more furniture was trucked to Florida, so now some of it would be coming back up north again, along with the cats. Moving was very expensive. Irene was depleting her meager resources.

Irene also missed the financial security and independence of being a police officer in Philadelphia. She had more than twelve years' seniority, which didn't give her much of a pension when she retired six months earlier, but it was a big step toward building a twenty- or twenty-five-year pension if she returned. And she loved police work.

It would be so nice—no more back and forth between Irene's house and my house, Philly and Florida. No more ring around the rosy. I got the vision in my head again of those "two against the world," but this time, I viewed them as traveling up Interstate 95 in a hurricane—heavy rain, thunder, and lightning—but with determined expressions and smiles on their faces as they anticipated their newest adventure.

Maria was wise enough to see that the southern move was not working out, and she and Irene were once again ready to commit, so they packed up. Irene left her Florida clan and drove back to Philly alone to my duplex.

Maria liked me a lot and was looking forward to talking to me. I loved listening to her, even though she was beginning to repeat herself just a little—probably no more than I do. I didn't mind hearing the same stories over again. The stories of her life that she retold were very interesting and extraordinary, and each version usually revealed a new tidbit. I always took notes, either in my head or with pen and paper—the old investigator in me, I guess. Maria smiled a lot and pointed to the legal pad I used to take notes, urging me to make sure I spelled "Skala" and "Stasurak" correctly.

I was doing the best I could to get a good picture of all Maria's relatives as she recalled her family in the Ukraine. I did some of the same searching for my own family and its Irish background—I found such investigations intriguing. By 2010, I put all Maria's information into Family Tree and printed it out. Her grandson had a frame made for it. The frame is about five feet wide. It's the only history that my in-laws have. It's still hanging in Maria's room in Bradenton.

Irene and I started looking for a house. In April 2003, Irene found a home, built in 1938, with a fieldstone fireplace in the living room and a formal dining room with a crystal chandelier. We bought it. She now had another project to work on. We painted the inside of the house from top to bottom. Always the industrious, energy-filled remodeler,

Irene placed plenty of doilies, draperies, and framed family photos throughout the house. She did the same at our Florida home.

On July 3, 2003, Irene flew to Florida and picked up Maria, who was staying at her other daughter's in Bradenton. Irene and Maria returned to our classic old home. Irene's mom was very happy to be with her "baby." Maria's bedroom started filling up with her own personal touches. She had her own bathroom too.

After we all settled into a routine and Maria was with us, Irene would smile and reach over to hold my hand. She'd tell me how contented she felt being with her mother and me.

"Tom, I've never been happier. I always hoped I'd find someone who loved me like you do. I have the two people I love most in the world right here beside me."

Irene just made me want to hug her all the time. "Honey, come closer."

Irene's taste in decorating our home drew many compliments from Philly neighbors, my sons, and other visitors. She loved Victorian, and our big stone home lent itself perfectly to that style. Irene also loved to cook. She introduced my sons to the flavors of goose and duck done in Old World style. They gobbled it up. During Irene's time with me and in her final days, she still enjoyed watching the Food Channel on TV more than any other.

By the way, Irene's cats came north with her, too. They were outdoor city cats. One survives to this day—Dusty. The other was hit by a car. Irene was difficult to console, for she found the mangled body herself in the street around the corner from our home. We went to a shelter and bought another one—the runt of the litter. We named him "Purry," because of his constant low purr. He was killed in the same street about a year later. Dusty never ventured far from the house. Later, Dusty was strictly an indoor cat at our Florida home. He stayed within the safety of the pool screen. That's why he is still alive.

Irene planted a small vegetable garden between our home and the one next door. We buried our cats in a far corner of the garden. That area is called a breezeway because of the wind-tunnel effect caused by the proximity of the houses. Irene always added her personal touch to her projects. Not one lazy bone existed in her body.

Whenever Irene went to the garden to harvest a vegetable or two, the tears usually filled her eyes. Irene wept quietly for several days. I did too. I loved what Irene loved. When Irene cried, I cried. Years later, when Irene didn't eat, I didn't eat. We both lost weight.

Who and what she loved, she loved deeply. I am so fortunate to have had the feeling of being loved unconditionally while she demanded nothing at all. What a rare characteristic. Her heart was so full. She often stopped me in stride, wrapped her arms around me, and whispered, "Thank you, Tom. I love you."

I wish I had done the same to her far more often than I did.

Officer Irene: Pre-Diagnosis

As soon as Irene returned to Philly in February 2003, we began the process of getting her back on duty as a police officer, maybe even a detective. She was reinstated on March 3, 2003, five months before being diagnosed with cancer. Prior to retiring in 2002, Irene placed sixty-seventh on the detectives' promotional eligibility list. That was higher than approximately twenty-five hundred candidates who competed on the exam. That was an excellent showing, an A++.

Irene was no dummy, and she had deep common sense, a necessary attribute for a detective. Further, while she was in retired status, the city promoted sixty-seven detectives. That meant if she had not retired, she would have been promoted, although as the last one of the first batch. That was just one other reason the southbound move was an unfortunate decision. But by returning, she had a right to be number one in the next batch. She would have to make that official request, which she did.

There was a lot of paperwork to complete her reinstatement. It took about a month, but she was finally sworn in again as a Philadelphia police officer. She then was assigned to a very busy district, the 25th, but that was fine with her. That was her first assignment when she graduated from the academy back in 1990.

Irene looked great in her uniform! And whatever she did, it was an all-out effort: being a cop, cooking, cleaning, washing a car, fixing her mother's hair, and loving me. She simply stopped at times, turned toward me, and gave me a hug. I wish I'd held her hand every moment we were together.

At times, Irene told me I had great legs—I don't, but she said it anyway. Sometimes she would flirtingly wink at me, always with that smile, and tell me I looked just like Clint Eastwood, Paul Newman, Brad Pitt, or someone else we'd just seen in a lead role in a movie. I don't look like any of them. But Irene, to me, was a knockout.

A few months later, she formally requested to be placed back on the official promotional list. If approved, she would be number one on the list. She composed the memorandum on July 10, 2003, before she was diagnosed with cancer. The memo was approved, and she was elated. She achieved one of her goals. She might get her coveted gold badge. In August, however, she was diagnosed with cancer which precluded a promotion. Ironically, on March 3, 2004, one year to the day after reinstatement, she was notified, along with several others on the promotional list, to report to the police academy for detective training. She actually had achieved only part of her goal; she would not be a detective.

Unfortunately, Irene was diagnosed in August 2003, with fourth-stage colon cancer. And although she fulfilled her responsibilities as a police officer once she was reinstated, she had to write another heartbreaking memorandum, declining the promotion. Writing that memo was one of the most disappointing moments Irene ever suffered.

Deep down, she knew it was going to be just a matter of time for other medical procedures in her treatment protocol. She felt as though she would not be able to work the extended overtime hours required of detectives in addition to coordinating future treatment regimens. Attention to her disease had to take preference.

In order to clarify the time lines so far, I'd like to remind you of the several events leading up to this point. Irene initially joined the Philly Police Department in 1990. After she graduated from the academy and received an initial assignment in the 25th District, Irene eventually was assigned to the 7th District, where she partnered with her close friend, our matchmaker, Sandy.

Irene spent a few years there and besides performing the normal duties of an officer, she often acted as an interpreter because the district had a large population of Eastern Europeans, mostly Russians. I wonder how her accent sounded to the listener as it was channeled through her Philly twang.

I met her for the very first time in 1999. Irene separated and divorced in 1999–2000. The second detective class she registered for was in 2001, after her divorce. She scored high on the exam as a result. We became an item after Sandy got us together in Atlantic City. In August 2002, she decided to retire and go to Florida with her mother to be closer to her immediate family.

Irene and I met regularly, up north and down south. I asked her to come back up north, stay with me, and get back on the Philly PD. She packed up and moved in by February 2003. We bought a house in April–May 2003, so we could bring her mother up north.

Incidentally, a week or so after we moved in, I slid down the steps from the second to the first floor on my behind. I installed a carpet runner from top to bottom and secured it with horizontal brass rods. In my stocking feet, I took the first step and then slid all the way down to a landing, where the staircase made a left turn. I knew Irene was the woman for me when I heard her scream and then came running toward me as I sprawled on the landing. She started to cry when she thought I was seriously hurt. I wasn't. But I saw the love in her eyes at the same time I saw the fear and tears. Irene was a person who could love deeply. She was definitely a keeper.

Irene got reinstated on March 3, 2003. She dusted off her uniform and shined her shoes. She hoped to be notified about being promoted to detective. Confident, Irene was as happy as she could be. Life was good, finally, for this struggling, energetic, smiling and very pretty woman. Life would be great for me too. It was a wonderful time for all of us.

But that sense of comfort was not going to last very long. In late July, Irene felt discomfort in her abdomen. She first noticed it in June but wasn't making a big deal about it. She had mild diarrhea, but she didn't want to jinx her recent return to the police department and potential promotion. A medical problem could have been unsettling at this time in her life and career. She was fretting quite a bit, though. I could tell. I strongly urged her to go to the doctor. I had my own history of ignoring pain with bad results. But Irene was not a complainer. She would let it pass. It concerned me.

It took a little coaxing to get her to make the appointment. I very gently threatened that I was going to put her bags on the porch if she didn't go to the doctor and have the pain diagnosed. She feigned fear, acting scared of me, with her ever-present smile, and promised to call her gynecologist in the morning. Neither of us expected what was to be in each other's future.

Irene called her gynecologist and made an appointment, as promised. She kept the appointment on August 7, 2003. Her doctor ordered a scan. The initial scan showed a 1.2 cm (about a half-inch) thickening spot on the right lobe of her liver. The images also revealed an area in the mid-sigmoid colon that was suspicious for cancer. Irene needed to get a colonoscopy—quickly. It was scheduled for August 19, 2003, twelve days later. We tried to pace ourselves. Of course, nothing is definite until biopsies are returned, we were told.

"Honey, it may just be fatty deposits. Please don't worry."

"Tom, what if it *is* cancer?"

I reached over to hold her hand. She always grasped mine, giving it a little squeeze each time.

It's hard for me to describe those horribly anxious twelve days between procedures. Irene was outwardly calm, as usual, but she confessed to me that she was frightened—very scared. Smiling, she downplayed the symptoms to anyone who asked. In truth, the only symptom was a pain in her abdomen. She thought, and hoped, it was just female trouble.

Her anxiety with regard to the colonoscopy, however, was evident. Subtle dread showed through her smile. We were hoping it was nothing, but what if it was cancer? Would her insurance cover the expenses? Did the break in her employment affect the coverage?

"Why now, Tom?" she asked. "Life is so good! It's never in my life been better!"

Irene's coverage as a police officer was second to none—her insurance would last as long as she was an active-duty officer and continue for five years after retirement. She used up some of the five years during her six-month hiatus, even though she had not been to a doctor in Florida. It was time that mattered, not doctor visits. But we wouldn't have to worry about that just yet. Besides, she was going to fight this thing and beat it, whatever it was.

We talked this way even before the colonoscopy and before biopsy results. We were both scared, hoping for the best. After all, many thickenings are simply fatty deposits, adhesions, or nonmalignant tumors. As long as they don't interfere with bodily functions, they can sometimes, depending on the size and location, just be monitored or removed with surgery.

Irene had a partial hysterectomy when she was younger, so we reasoned it might have something to do with removing her other female organs. Many women have that particular gynecological procedure and still live very long and active lives. Another disappointment for Irene was she never had any children. Very few women would be as great a mother as Irene would have been. She would have loved her children boundlessly.

Just prior to retirement in August 2002, Irene had a physical checkup with her family doctor. She requested a colonoscopy, but the doctor asked the usual questions and said it wasn't necessary—there was no evidence of cancer of any kind in her family, and she was younger than fifty years old (she was forty-nine years and nine months at that time). Given Irene's family history, there was no way of knowing, beyond her mother, father, and siblings, if there was cancer in the family. So Irene did not insist on the procedure.

We often think of what the results might have been if she'd received the colonoscopy in 2002. About a full year passed between that checkup and her first symptom, the abdominal pain. We wanted to believe that it was unlikely it would have made a huge difference. The disease probably had been growing for several years prior to her abdominal pain.

As another medical point of interest: I've had seven colonoscopies since my recovery from cancer in the '90s. At almost every other exam, I have polyps removed. I get them regularly. I had polyps cut out one year and had them again the next year. Polyps can be pre-cancerous, so I chose to get regular colonoscopies, especially since there was colon cancer in my family. I had relatives who fought and lost the battle. That was many years ago. I'm glad I knew of those relatives' illnesses. I tell my sons—do not wait past the age of forty to get the procedure!

08/19/2003: Colonoscopy today. Prep yesterday, worse than the procedure. To clean out, there is awful stuff to drink. The cleaning out is very uncomfortable. But it has to be done. Doctor could only go 25 cm (10 inches) into my sigmoid. He could not get past obstruction in my colon. He took biopsies. He suspects it may be cancer. He recommended that I have surgery as soon as possible.—Irene Stasurak

We received some bad news. The colonoscopy report did not conclusively say it was cancer. There was a very small, outside chance that it was diverticulitis with some perforation of Irene's colon. Nothing is certain until the biopsies confirm it. There was still hope. Everyone—friends and relatives—wanted to know the results of the lab report. We had to wait. Everyone was on pins and needles. We couldn't tell them anything, no matter how many times they called. Two very tense and nervous days went by.

Whenever we arrived in Florida, we described it: "Blue, white, and green—sky blue, clouds white, ground green." When we returned to Philadelphia, especially in the winter, we would comment, "Gray, black, and brown—gray sky, black clouds, ground brown." We were about to get hit by a personal storm of gigantic magnitude, a hurricane category five. The clouds were very dark and stormy and getting darker on that warm summer day at our home in the Fox Chase section of Philadelphia. And the storm was only just beginning to gather.

"Hold me, Tom. Please hold me."

I embraced the love of my life. We held each other close.

The Fourth-Stage Diagnosis: "Call Your Doctor"

Irene was walking a beat in a Safe Streets program on August 21, 2003, five months after rejoining the police department, when she was notified about the results of the biopsies. An operations room officer raised her on her portable radio: "Call your doctor." That was a tense few minutes before she was able to make contact.

08/21/2003: Oh, my! Biopsies confirmed my diagnosis of colon cancer. After colonoscopy at Nazareth Hospital, biopsies confirmed I was diagnosed with fourth-stage colon cancer (spread to liver through lymph system). Type: metastatic adenocarcinoma (big word, big trouble). Doctor arranged for colon resection at Nazareth Hospital, scheduled for next week, August 29.—I. Stasurak

She learned of the bad news while walking that beat, protecting the citizens of Philadelphia, who, when they saw and exchanged greetings with the smiling officer, knew nothing of her state of mind or the confirmation of her cancer diagnosis.

She called me right after she hung up from the doctor. I drove to her location in the 25th District—not a nice neighborhood. That was her very first district back in 1990. She was familiar with it. She was assigned there when she was reinstated back in March. When I arrived, she fell into my arms right there on the street, under the hot sun and in full summer uniform—handcuffs, Glock pistol, and all—with tears in her eyes. Passers-by just looked and said nothing. I convinced her to take the rest of the day off. She resisted at first. I drove her to the district to pick up her car, and she followed me home.

When we arrived at the home we'd just bought a few months before, we were in a daze. We went onto the shaded rear deck we'd recently decorated, just off the kitchen. We struggled with the reality of our situation through the tears. A neighbor passed by, walking her dog along the long driveway that ran the length of the city block. With a wave, she called out in the Philly twang, "How ya doin'?" Irene and I both gestured back to her and called, "Fine, thanks." We were anything but fine. The sun was going down, and the deck darkened. Irene's condition was beginning to sink into our minds. Our hearts were sinking too.

Questions abounded, naturally. What's going to happen? What about her job? Irene first wondered what would happen to her mother and me. That concerned her the most. How much sick time, holiday time, vacation time did she have available? Would it be enough? Would she be able to work during treatment?

After a restless, sleepless, and tearful night, Irene went to work the next day. If it was humanly possible, Irene would go to work. She was a great police representative to the community. The Philadelphia Police Department needs people with her professional attitude.

I followed her to those dangerous little streets in the Kensington neighborhood of Philly. I had a license to carry a firearm—or two. I walked along near my beautiful girlfriend, Irene. I wanted to know she was all right.

"Go home, Tom. I'll be all right."

"I love you. Remember that, honey."

I always told her I loved her on every occasion, no matter its nature, whenever we greeted or parted. I should have hugged her on those occasions more often than I did. August 29, 2003, the date for the colon surgery, seemed centuries into the future.

"Will they get it all?" she asked. "What about the tumor in the liver? Will they get it too? I want this stuff out of my body!"

We knew we were going to be peppered with questions from relatives and friends—questions that no one knew the answers to at that point. We'd been kicked in the teeth. In my mind, I kept silently urging,

Please, give us some space just now. Right now, it's all about Irene, not you!

Everyone was sincere in their concern, but when someone receives a diagnosis of fourth-stage cancer, his or her head is spinning. No one wanted to know answers more than Irene and me.

I was still running some seminars at this time, but I was distracted. Fortunately, I was near the finish line with them. I didn't say anything to anyone just yet.

Fourth stage—that was a shock. We educated ourselves regarding the various stages of colon cancer. Fourth stage of any cancer is usually indicated when cells from the primary tumor have worked their way through the lymph system into another organ.

In Irene's case, it went from the inside of the colon (first stage), penetrated the wall of the colon (second stage), broke out from the wall to the external portion of the colon invading the lymph system (third stage), and then spread through the lymph system to her liver (fourth stage). How could it be so pervasive? She was fine and looking forward to a splendid life and career. It was only a stomachache! There must be some mistake!

I went downstairs to my basement office and logged onto the Internet. The likely life expectancy for patients with fourth-stage colon cancer was probably two to five years under the very best circumstances, with the finest and most effective treatment. Zero chance of living beyond five years. I kept that information to myself. I didn't want to believe it. I refused to believe it. I vowed to rely on the doctors. We were going to place our trust in them from now on.

In the future, however, I would often use the Internet to look up definitions of drugs used in Irene's treatments and their side effects. Of course, each person's response to the various protocols is different. A person's body chemistry is very distinctive—not quite as definitive and specific as DNA or fingerprints but very individualistic. That's one of the reasons each component of blood workups has an acceptable range.

There are many different websites offering information to cancer patients and their caregivers. Anyone can Google any chemotherapy protocol and acquire information. We learned to have confidence in each of our medical team members at three different hospitals through the years. Irene always had the final word after the team's suggestions. We fought gloom and consciously made the choice to be positive.

When colon cancer is caught early enough—first, second, third, or even fourth-stage sometimes—it can be surgically removed and then followed up with chemotherapy, even if it goes to the liver, if that liver nodule is isolated. Maybe surgery can remove it. Life can be, at least, extended, as in Irene's case. We never gave up.

Radiation also is used in treating cancer. Of course, each progressive stage diminishes chances of effective treatment and the difficulty in medically handling all the complications. During my diagnosis and selection of treatment in 1990, I discovered some surgeons don't like to perform their art after radiation. The radiation has a tendency to char tissue a bit, which may obstruct the surgeon's ability to see all he or she needs to see. Irene wanted surgery. She wanted the disease out of her body. She reiterated that position several times through the years.

The moral of the story: get regular colonoscopy exams. The old saying is true: an ounce of prevention is worth a pound of cure. I hope none of us Cooney boys will need surgery or radiation.

The Battle Begins

I hope you know enough about Irene to appreciate how courageous she was and where that courage comes from.

It is impossible to adequately express what our lives were like and what a diagnosis of this disease does to a couple or a family. At the time, cancer completely occupies minds and hearts.

For the next eight years, ten and a half months, we lived to combat cancer and to squeeze any bit of enjoyment we could into our changed existence.

Lives do get turned upside down, but we trusted to the very end that quantity is quality. Irene and I believed that during the entire time of her suffering. Eventually, it was not a choice (either/or) between those quantity and quality; it was placing the two in the proper order.

Sometimes you hear friends and medical professionals prompting patients and their families to choose between the two, usually urging for quality. Irene and I understood that having someone to live *for* gives strength. It is the kind of strength police officers feel every day when they leave home for duty. They do what they have to do because they love their families and their families love them. Our love kept us together and gave Irene strength. I wanted desperately for Irene to live. Irene knew that. She was living and fighting for *us*. I'd waited my whole life for her, and I wanted to keep her. She wanted quantity from the doctors. Irene and I would provide the quality.

Caregivers should know why loved ones go through so much pain and agony in order to stay alive or at least to extend life. They need a reason to go suffer the torment of side effects. Love is what they seek.

It is because they can love so deeply. They do it for their survivors. In Irene's case, being the most unselfish woman I ever knew, equal to my mother, she battled for me and her own mother. Love enables mothers to struggle for their children; fathers also fight for their families as long as they believe they are loved. If someone diagnosed with cancer gives up without effort or little effort, I hope it is not because that person feels he has no one to live *for* or because she believes she is not loved. It was love that kept Irene fighting.

The only regrets Irene ever expressed to me were that she might not live long enough to take care of me in my old age and that she might pass away without being able to take care of Maria properly. Both responsibilities were extremely important to her. She was dedicated to Maria and me. It lent purpose to her life, she believed. Please, think about her dedication. That's what kept her going for almost nine years—she wanted to take care of us. When Irene thought of the possibility that she would die too soon, she always wept a little. She was always devoted to those she loved.

I tried to support her whenever I could. She needed encouragement. I would hold her hand and let her know she was not alone.

"I'm here, honey. We'll fight it together."

"I love you, Tom. I'm scared."

"I know, honey."

When I was free and Irene was off duty, we had dinner on occasion during that mind-bending week at a little family restaurant on Castor Avenue. In an effort to make light of the situation, she remarked that when I had Jell-O for dessert, I would swirl it and sift it through my teeth, just like she did. I thought everybody ate Jell-O that way. Irene assured me that we were the only ones in the world who did that. I tended to believe her. It felt good, true or not! She made me aware that I left sales tags on recently purchased clothing. So did she. Who knew that it was egg salad sandwiches, Jell-O, and sales tags that brought us together? We had so many habits in common. It was nice to believe it.

Irene ate salads, salads, and more salads. When we ate out, I had to coax her to get something that was, to my mind, more substantial. Invariably, it was pasta, fish, or chicken. She rarely ate red meat. She had calves liver—not beef liver—only twice that I can recall. She liked it. That was her diet for her entire adult life. She did not claim to be either a vegetarian or a vegan.

She reached across the dining table, saying, “Hold my hands, Tom.”

“Sure, honey.”

“I’m scared.”

“I know, honey. Don’t cry. I’m with you all the way.”

Colon Surgery: Updating Family and Friends

We held off most notifications of the families for a little while. We didn’t know enough yet. We thought we would wait until we had a lot more information about the disease itself and the prognosis. We were impatient to talk to the oncologists.

In the meantime, my sister’s oldest daughter had worked at the University of Pennsylvania Hospital. When she found out about Irene’s condition, she put in a call. She knew the director of colorectal oncology at Fox Chase Cancer Center, who had been at U of P at the same time as she was there.

I hand carried all the records, reports, film, slides, and scan results from Nazareth Hospital to Fox Chase Cancer Center. We soon were accepted into the FCCC program. The personal relationship my niece, Kathy, had with the director made Irene’s admission run smoother. Interestingly, Irene’s blood work at the time was perfect. No category was either high or low. It was all within the acceptable range. That changed drastically through the years.

The director remained personally involved with Irene’s case during every visit we made at FCCC for the following three years. After initial screening, the director always went over everything with us. But that was a little into the future. Irene still had a serious surgery to face.

08/29/2003: Surgery at Nazareth Hospital. Colon resection. Doctor will remove lesion in my liver if possible. Tom and I are praying.—I. S.

I floated for hours nearby in either the hall or the surgical waiting room while Irene was under the knife. The relatives knew that she was undergoing a major surgical procedure, of course. Everyone was calling me or the hospital, wanting to know Irene's condition.

They asked questions—Will this be all she needs? Will she be cancer-free after this operation? What are they going to do next? Is she out of the operating room yet? What's her room number? Why didn't you tell me what's going on? Don't you understand how much we love her?—and sometimes there would be the request, "Make sure you let us know exactly what's happening."

Picture me pacing in the hallway, waiting to hear from the surgeon, with cell phone to my ear, trying to field these questions coming from relatives who probably didn't know me all that well at that time. After all, I was that older guy from Philly who talked Irene into leaving Florida to go north and move in with him. In reality, I was scared half to death. I guess they weren't sure I loved Irene as much as they loved her and thought I wasn't as interested as they were in the outcome of the surgery. Trying to respond properly to all kinds of phone calls at such a moment was very taxing.

Many hours later, I finally felt relief! Irene had sustained the rigors of that very serious surgery and was in ICU. The surgeon, a pleasant middle-aged guy, sent a message to me with his wide smile, even before he spoke.

"Irene will recover nicely, Tom. It was very difficult. I got everything I could see. I wasn't able to reach that spot on her liver. That'll have to happen probably in about three months or so. In the meantime, she'll need chemotherapy."

Mixed in with my relief was the thought, *Good job, Doc! You did what you were called on to do. You got everything that was in her colon. You deserve your great reputation.* Preoccupied as I was, I didn't vocalize my praise to him, but I did sincerely thank him.

I was weak and barely suppressed an urge to cry. The pent up anxiety finally was released. Now I could fill in all those anxious relatives.

The cancer never reappeared in Irene's colon in all the subsequent years of scans. It reached her liver three additional times, the last time with pancreatic involvement. It would travel to her right lung, pancreas, and stomach as well but never in the colon again. Of course, at the end, it was very widespread throughout her whole midsection.

08/31/2003 (in ICU): Surgeon able to remove tumor in sigmoid (tennis-ball size), descending, transverse, and other scattered locations in colon (about eighteen inches total). He could not quite get to thickening in my liver. He also took out twelve lymph nodes from the area for biopsies. Tom here close by.—I. S.

I sat beside Irene's hospital bed and quietly watched her as she slept. It's so hard to witness a loved one in distress. You lose the normal composure that you can retain if you are not deeply in love. My lips were always close to a quiver. I touched her face and felt how overwhelming this situation must be for her. I remembered my own experience with the diagnosis of cancer. Yes, I remembered how concerned I was when I was in ICU after surgery.

As I watched her sleeping, I prayed she was not in pain and tried to send a comforting message through my thoughts as she slept.

Irene, I hope you dream pleasant dreams. We'll fight this, honey. Don't worry. And we'll be together doing it. We'll have many happy days, sugar, we will—you and me. Don't worry.

In future years, I would notice that her lips were on the verge of trembling and her eyes would fill up whenever we contemplated her condition. We did not avoid discussing her predicament—it was necessary—but we often chose to put it aside, just for a little while.

She spent more than two weeks in ICU at Nazareth Hospital in northeast Philly. The hospital is administered by Catholic nuns who run a tight ship, but I was always able to visit Irene, except under unusual circumstances, during the time she was there. Irene was subdued for a few days, but I swear I could see her smile, even though the nasal-gastro tube blocked a clear view of her mouth. It was taped to her nose going into her left nostril and down into her stomach.

Waiting for the lab reports made the days seem twice as long. The days and nights were uncomfortable too. Staying in the hospital is not a good way to spend time. The harsh tape on Irene's nose that was holding the NG tube in place was irritating the skin on her nostril.

Why don't the nurses use paper tape for that NG tube? I wondered.

Irene normally slept on her side, but she had to remain flat on her back. I know it was like torture for her, but she didn't complain. Trying to sleep and get comfortable caused the tape and tube to rub against her nose. Some nurses are better at taping down that tube than others. I manipulated it a little. That gave her some relief, but it really needed to be taped again or removed. I called the nurses, and they checked with the attending doctor. They removed it. which gave Irene a little bit of relief, but the skin on her nose was still a little raw after several days. I should have paid more attention.

There were many more tubes, drains, wires, and monitors attached to my loved one. Attached to her abdomen was a temporary colostomy bag. A Foley catheter hung on the side of the hospital bed. My heart was in my throat to see such a soul as Irene so encumbered. Hadn't she suffered enough in her life? Irene didn't deserve this—I hated cancer! During the first couple of days after the operation, I watched Irene's eyes open now and then, and then she smiled when she saw me. When she revived, the first words she mumbled were, "I love you, Tom."

That phrase seemed to be always on her mind, alert or not. It lifted my spirits, just as her smile always did. Can you understand how almost nine years of caregiving was effortless for me? I smiled and kissed Irene saying,

"Hi, beautiful."

"Hi, handsome," she whispered.

09/03/2003: Lab report: Seven of twelve lymph nodes were positive for disease. Biopsies confirmed lymph involvement. Doctor said chemo would be needed, as the disease is systemic. Tom and I will fight it together. I'm glad he's here with me. I'm glad we are together.—I. S.

Her ordeal at Nazareth Hospital, however, was not quite over. She had a pulmonary embolism, a blood clot in her right lung. Later, there would be a cancer nodule there.

09/04/2003: While still in Nazareth Hospital, I had pain in mid-back after colon surgery. Trouble breathing, too. CAT scan and x-ray confirmed a blood clot in right lower lobe of lungs. Heparin blood thinner administered. What else?—I. S.

Irene experienced at least three other episodes of clots in the years to come. Scared, I often rushed her to emergency rooms in nearby hospitals. After other surgeries, she was always watched carefully while in recovery.

Irene remained on some brand of blood thinner for the rest of her life. We took turns administering the needles. Giving Irene shots was no problem. Following my cancer surgery in 1990, I self-administered shots three times a week for a year. I used a Magic Marker to paint a tic-tac-toe design on each thigh and rotated through them to avoid inflammation at the puncture site. Irene and I developed a similar system, initially on her stomach and later, mostly on her legs, because of an increasing number of surgical scars on her abdomen.

09/05/2003: Family doctor visited. He seemed apologetic. I told him not to blame himself for any of this. My Tom came in later. Tom's here for hours every day.—I. S.

I missed the family doctor's visit to Irene that day. I never met him. He retired a couple years later.

Some days I was there a few hours, and some days I could stay longer, but I missed Irene every day. I ate lunch or dinner in the cafeteria. Through the years, I became very knowledgeable about the hospital food in both the cafeteria and in the rooms. I also knew of the off-campus locations where hospital staff went for their own meals. We were in a lot of hospitals. When I would dine in with Irene, we always enjoyed our bedside chats.

09/08/2003: MRI for liver. Maybe it's just a fatty deposit. Tom has a couple in his liver, he told me. They are common. He wants me to be positive. Keep hoping.—I. S.

Anticipation—nothing's for sure until the biopsies are returned; same goes for the results of MRI scans.

09/09/2003: Biopsies of liver lesion.—I. S.

09/10/2003: Biopsies positive for metastasis of colon cancer.—I. S.

"Well. It's for *sure* now, Tom."

"Yes, honey. But I'm with you. Don't worry, honey. I love you."

09/10/2003: They switched me to Coumadin and then lovenox. Better blood thinners.—I. S.

Some blood thinners are more expensive than others. Medical personnel prefer the more expensive ones for cancer patients. They seem to have a better effect, according to certain studies.

Later, after discharge from Nazareth Hospital, Irene needed a shot of blood thinner every day. The stomach area was recommended as an injection site in Irene's case, off to the side. Just put rubber gloves on, I was told, expel any air from the syringe, swab alcohol in an area, get a pinch of skin tissue between your thumb and index finger, push in with the needle, depress the plunger, withdraw the needle, and swab again. It was quick and painless—most of the time. Then discard the hypodermic in the Sharp's container. It was simple, easy. We could do that.

Through the years, however, we did have to inject in her thighs, too. A lot of very thick, surgery-related scar tissue and adhesions developed throughout her abdomen because of the additional operations she endured.

09/11/2003: Nurse changed the dressings again. Very big scar. Staples holding me together. They come out tomorrow. I may go home tomorrow.—I. S.

The incision was much bigger than that barely visible scar, faded from many years ago.

09/12/2003: Discharged from Nazareth Hospital; continue lovenox self-injections at home. Tom's good at it. Start process for acceptance at Fox Chase Cancer Center for Chemotherapy. I want to start.—I. S.

Hospital regulations require that a patient must be taken to the exit area in a wheelchair. This time and every other time, except toward the end, Irene attempted to refuse being wheeled out, but her attempts always failed. The discharge papers contained the usual instructions: no lifting over five pounds, no driving, take this and that prescription for pain, call if temperature goes above 101 degrees, continue self-injections, etc., etc., etc.

Relatives wanted to show how much they cared and that they were concerned. Irene was loved by all. I informed both our families and asked someone in each to be a contact so that I didn't have to go over everything each and every time another relative called. Of course, loved ones are concerned and if someone is not in the loop, feathers get ruffled. Neither caregiver nor patient wants to get into the middle of any brouhaha over "Why didn't you call me?" It is better, believe me, to keep the squabbles away from anyone going through such trauma. The appointed contact can spread the word and keep everyone informed. Irene's sister, Tammy, had that responsibility for Irene's Florida relatives. Sandy was perfect for this assignment among our friends within the police department. I handled my own family communications.

I was very grateful that communications eventually worked out. That is a big relief for those going through the distress. The caregiver can pick the time and place to fill in the contact relative or friend. But cell phone reception in hospitals is often very weak. Sometimes you get through and sometimes you don't. I was often in the hospital until very late at night. I also slept overnight on the cot that most hospitals have available for such situations.

After Irene was home for a few days, I changed the dressing. I used a 9x4 inch surgical pad. It barely covered her wound. There was a very slight half-inch curve at the very top, probably to avoid the umbilicus.

Irene was still smiling as she watched me at work, cleaning the area, applying the absorbent dressings, and being careful where and how I applied the paper tape. It made me smile too. This scar was going to leave a very large reminder.

Things seemed to settle down a little after Irene went back to work, and I continued whatever I was doing. We still looked forward to placing a port in Irene's upper chest so that chemo could be infused. The operation to attempt to get at the liver lesion was probably going to be in December 2003, as near as our surgeon at Nazareth Hospital could figure. That was a little more than three months away, but it would really depend on the schedules of oncologists and surgeons at Fox Chase Cancer Center. There was a lot to think and worry about in the interim.

One good thing—we lived about ten minutes from Fox Chase Cancer Center. Fortuitously, we bought our home near the very facility where Irene would later become a patient. Fox Chase is nationally recognized.

Through the years, we learned that it is extraordinarily important where a cancer patient is diagnosed and even more important, where she or he undergoes treatment. We had wonderful medical teams throughout our nine years of treatments.

Of course, Irene had to keep the police department informed of her condition. She wanted to get back to work. Irene always needed to be busy. When she did return, Irene was on "limited duty"—department-speak for inside work—while she fully recuperated.

When we had moments alone, we would try to make light of our situation.

"Looks like I'm going to be on the needle for the rest of my life, Tom."

"Don't worry, honey. I'll tell you I love you every time I inject you."

Irene would flash a broad smile, purse her lips, and return the jest.

"My, oh my, but aren't you the saucy one. Gimme hugs!"

⚜

Chapter Three

Infusion Port Insertion

10/07/2003: Fox Chase Cancer Center, pre-admission for infusion port insertion (relatively minor surgical procedure). It's just like it sounds. It's for access into my blood stream for chemotherapy.—I. S.

Publicly, we acted as if nothing was going on in our lives. The cats still needed feeding and their litter box changed. Meals had to be cooked and bills paid. Life went on.

Trying to act normally, we ordered a gas fireplace for my office downstairs in the basement. It was a fairly large area, carpeted, and furnished, but it was a little chilly in October and getting chillier.

A few blocks from the house was a factory outlet for all kinds of gas fireplaces. We bought one, and a friend installed it while we waited for news from Fox Chase Cancer Center. No one knew what our lives were like during that time.

People were very sincere in offering sympathy. But their lives went on. They worked, went to the movies or went shopping, and thought about what to buy or cook. Their lives remained on the same course. That was as it should have been. They thought about Irene and me and called, of course. Later, in Florida, with my sister's family nearby, they visited often, and we went to their home too. Visits were very uplifting for both Irene and me.

Irene and I went through motions automatically. Our minds were elsewhere. She still smiled. I still tried to. I wasn't quite the crooner I used to be when I drank two glasses of California red wine while stopping for a meal, driving on our trips south and back again. I quoted Shakespeare less frequently when I was in my cups.

The days were fewer when I sang along with Johnny Mathis's love tunes playing on the car CD, while Irene took over the wheel. Johnny was our favorite. His smooth, melodic voice put us in the mood as we cruised along Interstate 95. I would loop his CD—what person in love can listen to those ballads only once? We just had to hear it multiple times before allowing the CD player to move on to the next disc.

Hope springs eternal, as they say. My crooning days were not quite over, nor were my Shakespearean quotes.

Life continued. We still communicated with friends and family. We didn't withdraw. Neighbors visited and tried, in their way, to be uplifting. One well-meaning comment many people made when they heard of Irene's illness was, "You look great!" Please, don't take me the wrong way. I don't blame them, but such comments give little comfort. It's as if one can deny or ignore the entire diagnosis. Implied is "You look great, so that must mean you are fine. Ignore the prognosis, the surgeries, and the chemo sessions." It doesn't sound as good as intended to the ear of someone with fourth stage cancer.

Another common statement was "Call us if we can do anything." Think about that one. It transfers all the responsibility on to the people who probably are already burdened with chores and other things to do. Therefore, if the speaker doesn't hear from the needy person, the speaker is off the hook.

It's much more helpful to just do little things without being asked. Sometimes we listened to our answering machine when we returned from a twelve-hour day at the hospital in Tampa and heard this message: "Sorry we missed you. Give us a call if you need anything." Well, that caller was surely off the hook. His obligation was fulfilled. He called. Thanks a lot!

I would often be asked, "What can we do to help?" I would simply say, "Visit! Call, and ask if it's okay to come over." Just show up. Sit in on a five-hour chemo session or a ten-hour day with us, and go to the cafeteria with me when Irene tells us to take a break while she snoozes for a few hours in the lounge chair while getting her cocktail infused. Time! That's the greatest gift of love.

Visits and phone calls, most of the time, perked up Irene, as long as the visitors left their own troubles at home. Everyone was busy, we knew that. All anyone can do, really, is take valuable time to visit. That shows true love. Irene did get visits from many friends and relatives. It always uplifted her, even though she usually told them, "You didn't have to come but thanks."

But what is someone supposed to say? Probably something like, "I'm sorry to hear that. I'll keep you in my prayers." Mean it, and then resume a normal conversation. When such a statement is made in a sincere tone, it gives some comfort and an indication of understanding on some level. The speaker knows there is a serious battle looming in our lives. It's thoughtless to start relating the problems of others and especially mentioning all the friends who died of cancer.

For almost nine years, people told Irene how great she looked. Both of us, though, watched her slow deterioration in her once-beautiful skin and perfect figure. Irene was about five foot four and a normal weight of 130 pounds. Her weight, however, went up to 160 and down to 100 at the end. Her face thinned or rounded, depending on the chemo or steroidal prescriptions to counter side effects.

She used to say she was shrinking, too, getting shorter. She, in fact, lost about an inch in height over time. She kept her smile, and that made everyone overlook any physical decline. Through the years, I never let her know I saw subtle changes. She was still beautiful in my mind until the end.

10/14/2003: Per doctor's orders, switched back to Coumadin to be on the safe side for procedure tomorrow. Lovenox might thin blood too much. Don't want excessive bleeding.—I. S.

Almost a month after Irene was discharged from Nazareth Hospital, she finally received the phone call we'd been waiting for. She wanted to get started on ridding herself of the cancer in her liver. The director's office called and notified us to come to the Cancer Center for preadmission. Irene was scheduled for the insertion of the port in her upper-left chest.

Others have it placed on the right side. Irene was right-handed, so she chose, for no particular reason, opposite her strong side. Still others refuse the port and prefer to get chemo intravenously each time, either through the hand or arm. That works if only short term chemo is expected. But if chemo is to be long term, doctors recommend ports. Veins and arteries, over time, deteriorate with extensive chemotherapy. They are harder for nurses and technicians to find when other procedures, such as blood draws and scan preps, require it.

Later, it was difficult for nurses to find Irene's veins, just to get blood samples. The port came in handy at that time. The walls of her circulatory system became very thin and near collapse. But Irene's port survived the entire eight years, ten and a half months, even if her veins did not. At least one new style of port evolved and was prevalent—the smart port—as the years rolled on. As long as they are flushed regularly, lifespan is close to indefinite, I imagine.

10/15/2003: Procedure at Fox Chase Cancer Center: insertion of infusion port left upper chest. Will also see and schedule surgery appointment with doctor who will do liver surgery. He said to get some chemo in the meantime.—I. S.

Insertion of the port was an outpatient procedure. Irene was sedated, and the surgeon placed this ¾-inch thick by 1½-inch diameter device under her skin. It looks like a sixteenth-century snuff box. Once inserted, it protruded and raised the skin area on her chest a little bit. I read in the report that the insertion was a little problematic. The normal vein didn't lend itself perfectly for placement, but they were prepared and used another one that was close by. Irene's new port was an appliance most people don't have to deal with.

The port was accessed and de-accessed at each infusion, beginning and end. As years passed, and she lost so much weight, the port was much more prominent, pushing itself up and protruding under her skin. But after the procedure, Irene, trooper that she was, was back on the job right away, with her new port unnoticeable under her uniform shirt.

We just waited to schedule her first chemo sessions. We did not know exactly what to expect. But first, we met with the director. He determined the cocktail Irene would receive through her new port. That cocktail is not usually a *single* drug, even though that does sometimes happen. One is better than none.

Most often in Irene's case, they were combinations. The separate components of the cocktails had different functions. Part of it might kill cancer cells along with good cells, while another part of it isolated and starved cancer cells. Ideally, other drugs might interfere with the DNA of the cancer cells, preventing them from reproducing. They all aided in fighting cancer. Sometimes, Irene was given a sedative component with the dose to relax her, or other additives to combat expected side effects.

Often, the various combinations would be identified by acronyms—letters from each drug's spelling to shorten communication, both written and verbal. One example was FOLFOX, the acronym for the three drugs Irene received.

11/2003: Two visits in November with Director of Colorectal Oncology, Fox Chase Cancer Center, for follow-up after my colon surgery. He has a visiting Fellow assisting him also. Doctor prescribed weekly sessions of FOLFOX 6 (oxaliplatin, 5-FU and leucovorin).— I. S.

I'll describe these three components of Irene's cocktail simply to be representative of just one collection of drugs that she had administered during her years of infusions. Several other cancer-fighting chemo products from various pharmaceutical companies were available and were used in Irene's case to achieve the best effectiveness.

The specific type of cancer, the patient's height, weight, and endurance dictated what dosage was used. This was true regardless of the variety of cocktails. Control of side effects from oxaliplatin, for example, part of FOLFOX, became crucial with Irene. The dosages were decreased and ultimately discontinued entirely, due to Irene's eventual severe allergic reaction.

Oxaliplatin is a powerful and very effective regimen, but it gradually took its toll on Irene. It was the most effective, but at the same time, it had the most severe side effects. Earlier experience with it determined its value and its horrid side effects. It was finally discontinued when Irene went into shock during an infusion—more on that later. She knew it was dangerous for her, but she wanted "this disease out of my body." Ideally, oxaliplatin retards or prevents cancer cells from reproducing. Unfortunately, it does the same thing to healthy cells, including hair follicles. The good cells are eventually able to replenish, and the hair grows back.

Irene had extensive, severe side effects, but Oxaliplatin was very effective in both reducing and destroying various nodules that developed in Irene's system. It was used as long as possible, as long as Irene could tolerate it. She was very brave in confronting all that occurred.

Oxaliplatin is commonly used in colon cancer patients. The doctors always explained the various drugs to us. Oxaliplatin is one that interferes with the ability for the DNA of cancer cells to replicate themselves.

Irene had all the side-effects symptoms, to one extent or another, through all the years she was on chemotherapy. Some of the side effects were swelling, redness, numbness, tingling and cramping in Irene's hands and feet, and sensitivity to cold. Irene wore gloves when handling cold beverages or going in and out of the fridge. She didn't use ice in drinks and bundled up when going to and from the hospital, especially in winter in Philly. Nausea, vomiting, diarrhea, and fatigue were also common. It rarely went away completely—she experienced those side effects continually.

She also experienced mouth sores, difficulty eating and speaking, generalized pain in joints and muscles, low blood counts, shortness of breath, and—maybe the worst pain of all—anal fissures with diarrhea.

When FOLFOX chemo would start again, doctors had to eventually reduce dosage or skip it, because of Irene's severe reaction to the oxaliplatin. As the years went by, those symptoms never really left Irene.

Eventually, years later, Irene had an allergic reaction that required an emergency call in the infusion room. I briefly mentioned this scenario earlier. She couldn't breathe because her throat swelled, and she had to have oxygen to revive her. Of course, that reaction occurred in the most advantageous circumstances—in the hospital infusion room. After a week or so, she felt ok—that's what she said, but I could tell she was not back 100 percent.

The second component in Irene's first cocktail, 5-FU, is used in treating several types of cancers, including colon cancer. Its function is to help stop the growth of cancer cells. Diarrhea is one of its side effects, along with those associated with oxaliplatin. It is normally used together with leucovorin.

Leucovorin, in combination, helps 5-FU in its cancer-fighting activity and sometimes in reducing its side effects. It's not a cancer-fighting drug by itself.

I mention these three drugs at this time to give you an idea of the intention of the oncologists. Irene was treated at a research hospital with a very good reputation. By asking questions, we always were reassured she was getting the best and the latest cocktail. Irene would have her dosages changed several times during the coming years.

Reaction to chemotherapy has a lot to do with the patient's own determination, attitude, and philosophy toward life. Some patients refuse chemotherapy from the beginning, but Irene and I felt to do so was a very big mistake. We did understand, however, that some patients might want to forgo it and that there may be personal or even medical reasons (e.g., possible complications) to avoid the serious side effects.

Irene became very focused on her condition spiritually, too. She would often take her mother and me to mass. Irene always carried her rosaries and novenas with her. These aids provided a huge amount of comfort for her—I always hoped that it was so—because she handled the extraordinary pain and discomfort so well.

FOLFIRI and FUDR also are acronyms used together with other drugs. I always used the Internet to look up the acronyms, medications, and common side effects, so we had a better understanding of what to expect. The combinations of drugs seem endless. Of course, we knew Irene wouldn't necessarily have the same response as other patients to any treatment protocol.

Ongoing Chemotherapy and Ongoing Side Effects

Irene had a total of four chemotherapy sessions, spaced every other week, during the time between the colon and liver surgeries in 2003. They dubbed those cocktails FOLFOX 6. We did not know the name of each individual drug as they were delivered into her port sequentially. It consisted of oxaliplatin, FU-5, and leucovorin. Almost from the beginning, however, I got into the habit of asking the doctors and nurses for spellings, so I could look up the side effects and purpose of each drug.

The second session had to be delayed for a week because Irene's white blood cell count was low (known as *neutropenia*—one side effect of the oxaliplatin). She had to receive replacement units through her port before she could proceed. Low white cell count decreases the ability to fight infection. Infection would preclude getting chemo.

It caused us some concern. How careful did she have to be? How careful did I have to be? Did she have to go into seclusion? Should I wear a mask—that duckbill? Or should Irene? Should we warn everyone to stay away? I wish people would take the time to learn at least a little bit of what *not* to do if a relative is ill. I didn't want to be the cause of her catching cold or flu from me. We became anxious when a visitor got too close for too long. Would the medical staff determine Irene was unfit to continue? The doctors assured us and calmed our fears. They were great. First-time chemo infusions were often rough on the patient. Irene continued the scheduled sessions after that one-week delay, and the build-up of the white blood cells.

The sessions ran about four or five hours—basically, an hour or so for each drug and then an hour to recover. It was very convenient that we lived so close to the cancer center. That wouldn't be the case in Florida, later.

The sessions would deplete Irene, both during the drip and afterward. The crushing fatigue that resulted was different from and worse than normal fatigue. Irene would always bounce back, smiling, in those early days. She rarely missed work. She was provided with several prescriptions to combat the known side effects.

At any one time, for the rest of her life, Irene had to take more than fifteen different prescriptions as often as three or four times a day. Some helped reduce the side effects of her chemo infusions; some did not. They helped a little but never enough.

I kept a list of all the various side effects Irene suffered as a result of chemotherapy. It's a very long list, even though it's not complete. The list encompasses the usual nausea, vomiting, fatigue, overall malaise, and hair loss (alopecia).

In addition, Irene suffered through all the following, for both short and extended periods:

- painful, red, swollen fingertips and toes around the cuticles (paronychia);
- dry eyes (xerophthalmia);
- painful inflammation of any and all mucous membranes (mucositis);
- low white blood cell count (neutropenia), which diminished protection against infection and made Irene susceptible to colds or other communicable illnesses. She was hospitalized a couple of times so her white cell count could be replenished;
- difficulty swallowing (dysphagia);
- severe white yeast infection of the tongue (thrush);
- inflammation of the tongue, inside cheeks, lips, palate, and gums, making it difficult for her to speak, eat, and sleep (stomatitis);
- chemo-induced painful reddening, swelling, and numbness of the palms and feet soles (palmar plantar erythrodysesthesia, or PPE);
- severe shortness of breath (dyspnea);
- severe itching (pruritus);
- anemia and electrolyte loss due to diarrhea, vomiting, and related dehydration;
- very low levels of magnesium, requiring IV rehydration and supplements;
- very low levels of potassium, requiring IV rehydration and supplements; and last but not least,
- chronic pain.

Please note that this list is only the *physical* and not the *psychological* and *emotional* side effects Irene was suffering. The world of cancer is imperfect, as you can plainly see. She endured some or all of these side effects during most of the eight years, ten and a half months of her illness. The cracked lips, trouble forming words, and the visible white ulcers on both the sides and top of her tongue caused her serious discomfort. Eating and sleeping were difficult and painful. Our meals were meager during those episodes. No one really knew all that Irene was suffering; no one knew the emotional anguish. She didn't let them know.

At our next visit to Fox Chase Cancer Center for the chemo infusions, we learned that the liver surgery was scheduled for December 16, 2003. The surgeon's estimate was that Irene would spend about six days in the hospital and be recovered enough to be home for Christmas 2003.

In preparation for the liver surgery, Irene was given directions to discontinue any blood thinners two days prior to the scheduled operation. If her blood was too thin, it might result in too much blood loss during the procedure.

Irene was to be admitted for preparation on December 15, but in the meantime, she was to obtain scans and other diagnostic tests in anticipation of the surgery to remove the lesion that the initial scan discovered on August 7, 2003. We kept busy on her days off and when she was working second shift during that period.

Work-Related Schedules: Logistics

Irene didn't have to deal only with chemo. As with many cancer patients, she had to juggle treatment around work schedules. She had to accumulate time—sick days, vacation days, holidays, administrative days—as she would need time off in the future. It was a worry for us.

Fortunately, there was a provision in the rules that under certain circumstances, a police employee can go as deep as fifteen days in the hole, without pay, before he or she is taken off the books. Before Irene's first surgery, just in case, Irene had a "Request for Family Medical Leave of Absence" memorandum ready to submit to the police personnel department. We eventually accumulated all the necessary medical reports and documents. I helped her write it.

Irene had to forward the memo on September 2, 2003, after the colon surgery, as she had not accrued sufficient sick days during the recuperative period. It was close. She also had to pass a physical exam by the city doctors in the Health Department in order to return to work. She passed it and went back to work for a while in a limited-duty status, until she was eventually cleared for full duty. Irene was in that limited or restricted status a few more times before she retired in July 2006.

Irene's continuing to work did not mean she was feeling okay; in fact, she was feeling horrible. She just didn't complain outwardly. Irene religiously consumed the many prescription drugs to combat the side effects. She was supposed to be re-evaluated with an MRI scan prior to the liver surgery. Irene wanted to be in as good a shape as possible for the scan. She did not want anything to interfere with her treatment or surgery. Irene was very determined and looked forward to the operation. She wanted the operation to get the disease out of her body. Both of us were eager for her to have it. Imagine that—looking forward to major surgery!

We had a normal Thanksgiving—my sons came over with their dates. Amazingly, Irene and her mother, Maria, cooked a goose—Charles Dickens-style—with walnuts and cherries and all the fixin's. We bought the bird fresh at a market a few blocks away on Rising Sun Avenue. My sons and their girlfriends thought it was fabulous. The holiday came and went. Neighbors and family hardly knew anything was troubling us. Irene hardly missed any work during this time—very sturdy Ukrainian stock!

Inside the Fox Chase Infusion Room

We continued our weekly visits to the infusion room right up to shortly before the anticipated liver surgery.

The room was about 50 by 25 feet. The nurses' station was an island in the center. Very comfortable reclining chairs lined the walls, with patients' feet pointing toward the nurses' station, so that the medical staff easily can view everyone. There are a couple cubicles at either end of the room that, on occasion, a patient may get lucky and get a little more privacy during infusion. The cubicles also are used for special cases. Some patients who were very long into their extensive treatment were very weak and needed additional care. The cubicles provided just a little bit more privacy. Irene called them "the penthouses." Little did we know, she would need a penthouse, years later, during her treatment in Florida at another hospital.

At Fox Chase, every chair had a pump beside it on a telescopic pole. The device slowly administered the contents of each container of the prescribed chemo products. The pump defined, according to the prescription, the rate of flow over a particular time frame. Most patients had ports. The imprint of the port could be seen under their skin but when at home, at work or shopping, the port was inconspicuous under clothing.

In the infusion room, a nurse would prep and then install the access hypodermic lead into the port, the very center of which had a valve. The needle would penetrate the skin at the port site and the valve. The pump regulated the flow of liquid chemo into the vein to which the port was attached.

After finishing each chemo session, Irene drove to work—and she insisted on driving herself. She was glad she had a job indoors. She didn't moan or whine about her situation to anyone, nor did she play on anyone's sympathy. That was not—and never would be—Irene's style. As long as I knew Irene, she never complained publicly. Irene only mentioned her discomfort in the notes we both kept intermittently regarding certain treatments, surgeries, and hospital visits. Outwardly, Irene acted as though nothing was happening, but she would collapse when she got home.

We Christmas-shopped very early because Irene would be in the hospital on December 15 for liver surgery, the day after the MRI, and would be hospitalized about a week. We knew there wouldn't be a chance to shop later.

The malls were happy places and very busy. As we trudged through the crowds, I compared Irene's smiling face when she made a purchase to the clerk's returned smile. I saddened when I thought about Irene's suffering as we went about our daily activities. Thoughts would course through my head:

Why Irene? She doesn't deserve the pain she's going through. And she's so quiet about all her suffering—always smiling. It hurts so much to see her like this. She's not a whiner at all. Whiners do annoy me—those who are the center of their own universe; those who think they have bigger problems than anyone else. They are very vexing. Irene is the opposite of them.

Liver Surgery: Right Lobe Removed

12/16/2003: Doctor at Fox Chase Cancer Center surgically removed portion of right lobe of my liver (hepatic lobectomy). He also inserted external hepatic arterial pump to administer outpatient chemo over time directly into the remaining part of my liver. Uncomfortable wearing it. Something else to get used to.—I. S.

Irene spent more time in ICU with that darned NG tube again, chaffing the skin on her nose. I saw her every day. Nobody placed a time limit on me. I could stay at her side as long as I wanted. The food was a little better at Fox Chase Cancer Center than at Nazareth Hospital. Irene was recovering nicely, despite having to sleep while flat on her back with a Foley catheter and other tubes and wires coming out of and going into her body.

During this particular liver surgery, the doctor also removed her gall bladder and the remaining female organs, along with more lymph nodes, effectively helping to extend her life by eliminating a chance of disease in that adjacent area. Biopsies were always performed. I guess Irene's "change" was complete, hot flashes and all, after that surgery. In his surgical report, the doctor commented that the patient should be able to be home for Christmas and celebrate New Year's Eve. Her recovery would go well. He liked her and would see her a few more times in the surgical suite.

Another appliance for Irene to wear, the arterial pump, delivered a cocktail directly to Irene's liver: irinotecan, Avastin, and Erbitux. It was a different combination than her initial cocktail. No more oxaliplatin for now. That arterial pump was later removed after many months, but it was quite an inconvenience at the time to conceal it and protect it.

The pump itself was placed in a zippered canvas pouch. It was a cylindrical balloon-type device that held the pharmaceutical fluid. It was close to the size and shape of a household flashlight, maybe a little bit bigger. Traveling was more complicated, but Irene did get used to it, suffering just one more inconvenient apparatus.

I mentioned that Irene received Avastin and Erbitux in her cocktail. For a while, Avastin lost its approval by the FDA. We had a momentary problem with the insurance company over this drug. The carrier denied payment initially, stating that Avastin, in certain combinations, was experimental and so was not covered under Irene's plan.

We brought this issue to our team's attention, and they told us to forget about it. Eagerly, we did just that. Financial worries, at that time, were the last thing we needed. That was the last time we ever heard anything about it. Avastin was approved again by the FDA for certain chemo combinations treating specific type cancers, colon included.

Irene, as usual, made more friends as soon as she walked around the hospital ward. When she was able to walk, toting her IV fluid pump pole behind her and dragging feed lines and monitor in her wake, she visited other patients in their rooms. I accompanied her at times, when I was at the hospital. The other patients, doctors, and nurses loved her—and her smile.

The liver surgeon was very protective of Irene and demanding of the nursing staff, ensuring Irene had the proper care in ICU and in her room on the normal hospital floor. The nurses said he was grumpy, but if they had to have surgery, he was the one they wanted to perform it.

12/22/2003: Discharged (Dilaudid and Coumadin to be continued for five days at home). I bid everyone good-bye. Wheelchair again; Tom is driving it.—I. S.

Irene would be on Dilaudid for the rest of her life, along with several other standard side-effect reducers. We relocated to Florida in 2006, and that would cause a big problem in 2011, when she ran out of it, though only briefly. Dilaudid is a painkiller, a derivative of morphine. That was two days of severe hardship for Irene—withdrawal. The withdrawal is exactly as portrayed on TV: brutal, accompanied by screams, sweat, and tears. Dilaudid is very addictive and by that time, the dosage was large. We called the physician's assistant at the hospital in Florida when we realized Irene was going to run out of pills. The PA had to mail us the prescription after approval by the doctor. Narcotics can't be simply called in. Irene went those couple of days without her painkillers. We were much more careful from that particular time forward in pacing her usage.

Over the next several years, I became very friendly with the pharmacists at the Acme Supermarket around the corner from our home in Philly and at Publix Food Market, ten minutes away, when we were in Florida. I made many, many visits to their drop-off and pick-up counters for Irene's prescriptions. I think the pharmacists miss Irene and my talking about her. They always asked how she was doing. They felt as though they knew her.

At home, the numbness in her hands, the fatigue, nausea, and diarrhea, plus the hot flashes did not erase her smile. Irene raised her eyebrows:

"Whew! It's hot in here, Tom."

It took me a few seconds to catch on to Irene's comment.

"Wow, honey. It's December! Oh, I think I know what you mean. I'll turn down the thermostat a little. Do you want to sit out back for a little while? It's chilly."

"I think that would be nice. Just for a few minutes. Thank you, dear."

Home for the Holidays

Christmastime, with all the bells and whistles, was alive and well at our twin home in the Fox Chase section of Philadelphia. Irene would have it no other way. Lights and wreaths and mistletoe were scattered throughout the house.

Visitors were very complimentary on what a great job Irene did with decorating the house along Victorian lines (two opposing loveseats, complete with doilies, perpendicular to the fireplace in the living room), as well as her flair for holiday ornaments. The live tree was fabulous and took up a good portion of the living room. It was topped with an angel and my touch—a Christmas ball with a picture of my sons on it. Visitors hardly noticed Irene's exterior arterial pump.

My sons and their girlfriends had duck with orange sauce and all the trimmings for the first time that Christmas. After dinner, they continued their frolicking and visiting to their various other relatives. We made the phone calls to Florida to inform Irene's siblings that everything was going well and to extend holiday greetings in a timely way, to catch everyone at one location, at her sister's place. On the surface, all was well.

When people left and we were alone, we hugged and sometimes wept a little. People continued to "encourage" us with words like, "Things are different today. It's not as big a deal as it used to be." *Really?* I thought. *You just don't know. Your life has not been affected.*

Worse yet was when people asked Irene how she was doing, and Irene would begin to comment, thinking the questioner was actually interested. Then, that person would drift into an explanation of what he or she went through during an episode of chicken pox or whatever. Irene and I called this type of conversation the "segue."

In the "segue," the talker was only interested in telling us about his or her own problems. Irene and I would look at each other and smile as the other person kept on talking.

A similar type of conversation was the "sidebar." Someone would ask Irene how she was doing; Irene would tell the person about her latest scan; and then the questioner would look away from Irene and respond to a piece of conversation he overheard elsewhere in the room. Irene would just walk away from that person, as she was no longer part of that conversation.

Life Goes On: We Hope

I had a doctor's appointment myself in late December 2003. I was informed that I passed the line from being pre-diabetic to full-blown diabetic and that I also had high blood pressure. Over the last several years, I had put on some weight, reaching 190 pounds. (Ideally, I should be about 160 pounds, which is what I am now.)

My God, what next?

I was put on meds for both conditions. I had always been a runner and a jogger, and then a fast walker, and then simply a walker. Irene got my running shoes out of the closet and barked an order.

"Hit the park, handsome,"

"Okay, hon. Gimme a hug and kiss first, just in case I keel over."

Irene frowned at my attempt to joke in order to get a hug and a kiss.

"Tom, please don't say that. I need you around me."

I hit the park. But it was winter! She made me bundle up and drove me to one of the entrances to Pennypack Park. You could do ten miles or more in there, if you wanted to. Eight was my limit at this time. I didn't want to be gone too long, and every mile took longer as time went by. I'd call her when I was pooped and ready to come home.

I started trimming down as the cold weather really started hitting the northeastern United States. Irene urged me to cut down on carbs, milkshakes, banana splits, pie, and other desserts, all of which she saw me consume at one time or another. She laid out my daily menu and walking schedule. She was as interested in my health as I was interested in hers.

We both knew we had to depend on each other. No one else would take the extraordinary effort we needed for each other. Irene and I were bound together. My problems were simple to control. Controlling her illness would not be as easy.

Once, after I overdid it in the park, I came home, and my beard was full of ice. I went upstairs and collapsed on the bed. She took off my shoes and the rest of my clothing while telling me she loved me and then made me some hot chocolate with whipped cream. No carbs in the whipped cream. She made the hot chocolate with water. Typical—Irene, the caregiver.

What Does the Future Hold?

Yet there was hope. There was a chance, according to our medical team and the report from the surgeon, that the liver lesion might have been isolated and that chemo might prevent further spreading of the cancer to other organs through the lymph system. Now that the tumors had been cut out of the liver and the colon, we were *only* dealing with the disease in the lymph system. Maybe—just maybe—the new cocktail would eradicate them.

There was hope—but there was a lot of false hope, too, when we searched the Internet for "cures." It was interesting how many people wanted to provide information they'd just discovered on a website in Canada, or Germany, or wherever. But this was life or death for us (not so for them). Besides, we couldn't mix remedies. Which treatment would we praise or blame if Irene got better or worse? And there was no scientist in the Ukraine, as Maria heard through her grapevine, who had developed the cure for cancer but was not allowed to distribute it because of government control. Maria was hoping and praying, too.

Oncologists who know their field can give direction, and they are aware of the very latest procedures and drugs, especially at research facilities. We stuck with them. We lasted almost nine years after a diagnosis of fourth-stage colon cancer. I think that proves we charted the right course.

Irene and I stayed home on New Year's Eve. We were not in the mood to be driving among the drunks. It wasn't our style to drown our troubles in booze. At this time in our lives, we enjoyed a couple of glasses of wine or a couple of mixed drinks—one or the other. We were not being stereotypical Irish or Ukrainian! We didn't go gloomy, but we did want to be alone. We stayed close to each other.

We would always try to cheer each other in different ways.

"Gimme a big kiss, handsome."

"Glad to oblige, Scarlet."

Our love for each other came through. We hugged and held hands a lot. I'm so glad today we had that closeness between us. We were going to be pretty much alone, geographically and emotionally, within the deep trenches of this battle.

We discussed what our next course would be. The doctors planned to resume chemo after the liver surgery. We would meet with them early in January, after the holidays. We started talking about possible trips we could take. At first, after the diagnosis, we had a little anger but it was brief—anger was a waste of time. We moved on to "We'll fight."

We wanted to get back to normal as soon as we could, even though we didn't know if that would ever happen.

I started thinking about wrapping up my business so, if needed, I could be available full time for Irene. It was too soon at that point, but thank God I was in a position to do so.

As it was, I arranged my seminars and any other duties around Irene's doctor and hospital visits. We were fortunate in that regard. We also didn't have to worry about medical insurance coverage at that time or that our income and assets were dwindling to nothing.

We smiled at times when we heard Irene's family, my sons, or others tell us about some good fortune they'd had, such as business was good or how nice their new girlfriends were.

Other times, our smiles would be muted. There never was a more eventful year than 2003 and now we would face a new year with new hurdles to jump and bridges to cross. We got ready for it. We were looking forward to moving along. We stayed home on New Year's Eve.

"Happy New Year, honey!"

"Let's celebrate, Tom. Break out a bottle of Shiraz. No! Let's bring a bottle of Beringer upstairs with us and watch the New Year come in."

In 2004, there would be a few complications with Irene's treatment. That direct line delivery of irinotecan, bevacizumab (brand name Avastin), and cetuximab (brand name Erbitux) would cause her a lot of distress. But it would not incapacitate her. It takes much more than that to knock her down. We also did quite a bit of traveling to take the edges off. Our little conversations supported both of us.

We liked to sit on the side porch of our house in Philly and sip a glass of wine. Some of the most important conversations we ever had occurred on that porch along with some of the most humorous.

Irene always looked so beautiful. One evening, the moon struck her smooth skin making it glow as we sat on the porch glider. I always wanted to ensure Irene knew I loved her. It was important for her to know that.

"I'll always be here for you, honey."

Irene flashed that gorgeous smile and reached for my hand. When she held my hand she squeezed it as usual.

“I know, Tom. It’s you and me. I wouldn’t trade my life with anyone right now.”

Her response triggered a vague memory:

“For thy sweet love remember’d such wealth brings; That then I scorn to change my state with kings.”

Wide-eyed, Irene looked at me quizzically and commented softly,

“That’s beautiful, Tom. Who said that?”

I took a sip of wine, swirled the glass a little and answered,

“That was Shakespeare, honey. I’ll do the whole sonnet for you one of these days. You’ll like it. And it expresses exactly my feelings about our relationship from the first time we got together.”

“I can’t wait, Tom. Please tell me now.”

I felt a little lightheaded from the wine which put me in a playful mood.

“I can’t. I have to re-remember it.”

“Re-remember it? Are you speaking in tongues, Tom?”

I leaned back on the glider and planted my feet so I could create a little back and forth swinging motion.

“You talk about remembering, honey. Remember that time when we were skinny-dipping in the pool and the heron landed on the screen? That big bird turned around right away, stared down at you, and let loose a load. He was telling you something, honey.”

Irene giggled a little.

“No, Tom. He was staring down at you when he let loose. He hardly knew me. I hadn’t really chased him before that. He was telling *you* something.”

"No. He was saying he didn't care if there were two of us now. He was gonna do what he was gonna do—doo-doo!. He'll do doo-doo."

We both took sips from our wine glasses, held hands and relaxed. We put aside our cares for the moment. We waved at passing neighbors we hardly knew—but we waved to them anyway and they waved back. It was a friendly neighborhood.

Irene and I went back and forth for a little while. I reminded her that the big blue heron got tired of us quickly that particular day, I think. He just flew away with a final over-the-wing glance back at us, implying he would be back. He came to do something when he heard us in the pool. He did it. Then he just departed, having deposited his message for both of us.

That incident with the blue heron that Irene and I recalled happened in late 2002. It was during one of Irene's early visits, while she was still living in Bradenton, Florida, after she initially retired from the police department.

The "Heron War" continued year after year, all the way up to the day Irene's soul left this world and went on into the next. Then, under some unusual circumstances, something strange happened that has continued to this day.

Why hasn't the blue heron come back, Irene? Was that you?

⚜

Chapter Four

There's More to Life than Chemo and Surgeries

Well, 2004 arrived, and we readied ourselves for whatever it had to offer. Chemo was still dispensing through the arterial pump from the time it was inserted until it was removed in October 2004, after ten months. During 2004 and 2005, Irene would have nine blood draws during visits to Fox Chase. One concern of the medical team was the level of CEAs.

CEA (carcino-embryonic antigen) is basically a tumor marker in colorectal cancer patients who've had surgery. It's an indicator in much the same way that PSA (prostate-specific antigen) is a marker for prostate cancer. The team wanted to make sure there were no recurrences of the cancer over an extended period. The markers were closely watched. Elevated levels signaled danger. Irene was within the expected range during this time.

01/2004: The external pump installed during my liver surgery was still active. The chemical was called irinotecan, among others, which, in response to my body temperature, would release directly into my liver. I think one month irinotecan plus the others; one month saline solution. Will exchange it regularly. Difficult to get used to this purse-sized thing attached to my side. So what? Tom still loves me, though.—I. S.

"Irene-tecan." The drug was named after Irene! The doctor pronounced it that way intentionally so he could see Irene's eyes and her smile widen. That seemed to be a good omen. The real name is irinotecan.

Irinotecan is used mainly in metastatic colon cancer, that is, when the disease has already spread. This drug actually interferes with the growth of cancer cells but while it's killing them, it can kill normal cells too. Like oxaliplatin, it can cause hair loss—the least of a cancer patient's troubles when all things are considered but which often causes the most heartache among women. Irene continued losing her hair.

Irene always had a beautiful, thick head of hair. When she started losing it, we were told, "It always grows back." And it did, but it wasn't the same. It went through a "rabbit fur" stage and was a little frizzy. A wig solved that problem. We bought one, but Irene wore it once. The weather was getting warmer, and it was uncomfortable. Irene quickly adjusted. She switched to a baseball cap. She lost the hair all over her body a couple more times before it was all over. She raised her sparse eyebrows and widened her eyes whenever she told that to anyone. Eventually, it grew back. She looked so cute in that cap. It was green and had a gold shamrock on the front—Notre Dame. I still have it. Still, trouble brewed—a blood clot.

02/16/2004: Tom rushed me to the emergency room at Jeanes Hospital. Very close by. It is located right next to Fox Chase CC. My right lower leg had swollen. A scan in the ER easily spotted a blood clot. Clots are more common in cancer patients. Blood thinners were prescribed, and we went right next door to FCCC and had a Greenfield filter placed in my groin to prevent clot from traveling to my heart. Very, very dangerous if that happens.—I. S.

We were told to make sure we reminded our oncology team at FCCC to schedule the Greenfield's removal in no longer than two months. The doctor who placed it was from the surgical department, and it was after hours. If they didn't get it out within that time frame, it would have a tendency to get entangled in new veins and arteries that the body generated, trying to make their way around the foreign object.

04/2004: I had a mammogram done. No suspicious activity. One less worry.—I. S.

04/2004: Surgeon could not remove the Greenfield filter. Too congested with new growths. He didn't want to risk tearing the femoral artery. I could have bled out.—I. S.

Irene was recovering from the sedation, and when she was alert, I told her the news. It was another disappointment, but it was better than Irene's bleeding to death on the operating room table.

The filter was never removed—and that, as it turned out, was a good thing. She suffered more leg clots in the future, and the filter continued doing its job, even though it got very messy inside her right lower groin area, we discovered later.

The arterial roadblock would cause a physician's assistant some difficulty a few years into the future. Irene qualified for a certain immunotherapy program that required a catheter placement through one of the femoral arteries, the big ones in both sides of the groin. The normal route was up the right side. I told the PA about the Greenfield, but he said he'd done a thousand of these procedures and wouldn't have any trouble. He started—and Irene screamed.

Irene had a very high tolerance for pain but as he continued to thrust the catheter, Irene screamed again. He reinserted it in the left femoral and it went smoothly. It was a different route than normal, but it achieved its purpose. He apologized, and Irene accepted the apology. I didn't.

Other medical personnel over the years often deferred to our recollection of treatments from the past. They wanted the best information. They at least considered anything Irene and I could add to their collection of information. I can still hear Irene's screams to this day. I get a little chill as I sit here and reminisce.

Some Time to Travel: Let's Enjoy

Even though the pouch was cumbersome, we decided we could travel. If we thought it necessary, Irene could have the arterial pump disconnected for a while during the saline solution phase of the pump's delivery system. We believed Irene should not take a plane anywhere, due to the temperature and pressure-activated nature of the arterial pump. The surgeon who placed it made himself available whenever we wanted to take a flight somewhere, or even if we were just driving to Florida to visit relatives and returning. He was great. We took advantage a couple of times.

Irene was very well recuperated from the surgical procedures she'd endured over the last several months. She still had that nagging fatigue, nausea, and tingling in her fingers and toes, but she told me she felt well enough to head south or to fly somewhere. She was a trooper. And she wanted to give me some relief from the intensity of the past seven or eight months. We both needed a short release.

Irene was still on limited duty, and no one at work commented on the pump. It didn't interfere with her responsibilities, and coworkers were used to it. A few of them were also on limited duty and had issues of their own. Those officers and civilian personnel hardly noticed that bulge under Irene's clothes anymore.

I was on my own self-imposed limited duty. I was winding down my business. I didn't announce any new seminars, and I didn't take on any consultations. The timing seemed to be good because it was in between the city's promotional exam announcements. I was as free as I wanted to be. And I was eager for Irene and me to get away from it all. We got the pump temporarily disconnected.

California Wine Country

We decided to go west! It would be a great getaway. We promised to hardly speak of cancer the entire time. We used air miles I had accumulated through the years. If I ran out, I could count on using buddy passes through my sister's youngest daughter, Maureen, who was a stewardess for a major airline, but I had loads of air miles.

We combined a couple days with Irene's regular two days off work, one on each side, giving us four days. We were interested in enjoyment and freedom from the aggravation and trivialities of daily life.

We continued in our status, treatment break, as the doctors called it. Liberation! Irene went to work every day and racked up enough leave time. We needed it in the future too. But a vacation was in order. We, of course, were ready.

Irene had a nephew in northern California. We would make it a two-fer. We could visit Irene's nephew and his family and then visit several wineries before we returned to Philly. We would drive over the Golden Gate Bridge on our way to Napa Valley.

We landed in San Francisco, spent a day there at the wharf, and then drove up and down those steep streets. It was scary when I couldn't see anything but the sky through the front windshield, when I leveled off at each intersection, as we drove downward. Irene let out her favorite exclamatory yell once or twice.

"Whoopee! Whoopee!"

We were having fun. Then we drove our rented car to Napa Valley, soaking up the sun in that chilly area and took in the beautiful scenery on the way. When we crossed the windy Golden Gate Bridge, we could see Alcatraz. We traveled through the champagne country, taking pictures of the different vineyard's castles. We arrived in Napa earlier enough to go to a tasting at Beringer's winery, one of our favorites. Then we settled in at a very picturesque Thomas Kinkaid-type bed-and-breakfast we'd booked before we left home.

We wine-tasted at the wineries from the bottom of the valley to the top and then returned in the opposite direction, doing the same thing. I had been there before, but it was the first time for Irene. It was wonderful to see Irene experience something for the first time—eyes big and the smile bigger, like a young child. She loved it. I loved it too, because I was able to see her loving it.

We were cautious wine tasters. It was easy. They don't give us much wine. I guess that's why they call it a tasting. We went to the most famous and popular vineyards. All of them had magnificent vistas overlooking the slopes, undulating across the rolling hills, down and away from the gorgeous castles and mansions. We joined a couple of full tours of the wineries and visited Irene's nephew and his wife and two sons as well. They eventually moved to Bradenton, Florida, by the way, to be closer to his parents and family.

But we didn't have any more time. Irene had to get back to work. We purchased several bottles of wine and brought them onto the plane with us. The plane was half empty. We started a conversation with a wearied flight attendant. It was a turnaround for her on her second six-hour trip. She'd finished her duties for the present. When she saw that our carry-on was chock-full of Napa's best, she gave us a corkscrew. We were having fun, and so was the flight attendant, as we sat, laughed, drank, and conversed in the back of the plane. The flight landed in Philly before we knew it. The trip was one of the best respites we had since Irene was diagnosed in August 2003.

Irene was reunited with the arterial pump, but we were not quite done taking advantage of the break from hospital infusions. The steady irinotecan drip directly into Irene's liver did take a toll, however. We couldn't wait for the next phase of saline solution replacement.

A few months later, we were free again, thanks to our friend, Dr. Grumpy. We really loved him. He wanted us to get quality along with the quantity. He believed, as we did, that quantity, with its potential for new discoveries and surgical procedures, along with pleasure, would provide its own quality of life.

A Short Trip to Vegas

Off we went again, tying in two vacation days with Irene's regular two days off. This time, it was Las Vegas. Cirque du Soleil's *La Nouba* was bringing in record audiences. I reserved plane tickets using air miles again, and we flew west. My niece, Kathy, arranged for us to stay in a beautiful time-share on the Strip. She has some very good connections. It pays to network.

We walked the Strip, took in some shows, and did a self-directed hotel tour: Caesar's, Treasure Island, MGM, New York New York, the Luxor, and a few others. Taking in the lobbies and spectacles of those grand hotels was worth the effort.

I reveled in seeing Irene's glee when she did something for the first time. Her smile broadened even more than usual—she seemed to be a young girl again. It was charming and brought a wonderful feeling into my heart to watch her take it all in, with a very contented smile on that pretty face. Her life's experiences had not exposed her to the sights she was absorbing.

Irene was feeling the usual side effects, but she ignored her discomfort and pain. She wanted to play some slots, and we won a few dollars, but gave it back at the airport, waiting for our return flight. Doesn't everyone who goes to Vegas do that?

We carried a heavy burden, but we both smiled all the time, and whistled in tune with each other—that made a big difference.

The Sunshine State

In late summer, our little suburb near Orlando was hit with three very destructive hurricanes. In August 2004, a year after Irene's diagnosis, we flew to Florida to visit relatives on both sides. We took a plane rather than drive so we could spend more time. It is only a two-hour flight. Several years later, Irene wouldn't be able to endure any amount of flight time. We took advantage. Irene did the usual—she added a day before and a day after her two regular days off. Her superiors were glad to authorize it.

A sufficient number of officers in limited-duty status always are available to cover any responsibilities. They were either facing a medical condition themselves or were injured on duty and not yet a 100 percent. An officer had to be 100 percent physically fit and approved by the city medical office in order to return to full duty. Safety was a major concern throughout the organization. The PPD was an eight-thousand–member force at the time, in a very busy city, from a law enforcement point of view. There was always plenty of sickness and numerous injuries in a city police force that handled more than three million calls a year into the dispatch center.

I had another car in Florida, so we drove to the west coast in two hours to see Irene's relatives. The drive was tough on Irene, but she wanted to see her family. Her mother always encouraged us to enjoy ourselves. Maria would be fine up north, and Irene's family in Bucks County was close by, just in case. We wouldn't be gone long.

When we made the trip across Florida to Bradenton, Irene would get in the car and immediately recline the passenger seat all the way, close her eyes, and try to rest. She always apologized to me for doing that. I told her there was no need to apologize. She apologized every time anyway. As we approached Bradenton, she brought the seat back to normal and sat up.

In that same sentiment, whenever I drove her anywhere, when we arrived home and pulled into the garage, she always said, "Thank you for taking me to the hospital" (or store or mall or Bradenton). We had almost nine years of doctor's appointments. I was never inconvenienced by any of those trips. I told everyone that my caring for Irene during her illness was effortless. It was not inconvenient in any way. It was a privilege. It was a privilege to love her and be loved by her. I loved Irene.

As for my family, it was only a twenty-minute drive from our Florida home. Everyone was glad to see us, and we had a great time visiting. Everyone unanimously agreed that Irene looked great. They always said that. They wanted, in their way, to make her feel good and try to encourage her to ignore or deny her condition, at least for a little while. Irene would say thank you, naturally.

Irene suffered but kept it to herself. Irene was still very active, and she participated in any activity wholeheartedly. At my sister's, we played games like Trivial Pursuit. We sat out back on their lanai, watching the sunset and always had a good time. Family is a key ingredient during any hardship.

From the initial diagnosis in August 2003, to our trips in the wine country and Vegas seemed like a hundred years. We climbed Mount Everest, crossed the Gobi Desert, and walked a tightrope over Niagara Falls. We could handle more chemo when we must—and even hurricanes!

On August 13, 2004, we had a visitor. His name was Charley. A category 2, he came across our little town, blowing at 105 miles per hour. The rain and wind sounded like the locomotive everyone talks about when describing hurricanes and tornadoes.

My house had single-pane windows—certainly not good enough to withstand 105 mph winds. We just hoped the panes wouldn't give way. Our windows didn't break, but they still let in a lot of wind-driven rainwater—the wind just bends the glass. Codes have changed quite a bit since then. In 2009 and 2010, I upgraded the windows and put on a new roof after being tired of years of continuous repairs that never quite solved the problem.

There had been no hurricanes in Central Florida for seventy-five years. Hardly anyone watched the Weather Channel—no need to. The weather was always good. The sun always shined brightly. It rained at 4:00 PM, stopped at 5:00 PM, and then cleared, almost the whole summer. Winter, the dry season, was perfect weather—the reason people move to Florida.

When Charley hit, Irene and I watched our pool screen get ripped out of the ground and tossed onto the next door neighbor's property, along with all the patio furniture. Both of us were insanely trying to keep the sliding doors to the lanai from crashing in by leaning against them—we were ignorant city people. We ran upstairs with arms full of towels trying to soak up the water coming in through the second floor windows. It soaked the carpeting and seeped through onto the downstairs ceiling.

Thank goodness, we were only without electric power for about five hours, after which we could run the dryer. All the electric is underground. This northern boy didn't have a generator. It was a running battle between the dryer, the windowsills, and floors, and constantly drying and re-drying the towels, even though we had at least three dozen of them. Irene had to be careful to protect the arterial pump all the time, too, as she scurried to and fro'.

The same thing was happening on the first floor. The pool was overflowing and threatening an invasion but the drainage system was good enough to prevent that. We abandoned the sliding glass doors and headed for the bathtub. We stayed there until we got the all clear. The next day, we found our barbecue grill in the street out front. What a mess! It was Friday the thirteenth, by the way. Strangely, it was exciting.

We had reservations to fly back to Philly, but I stayed behind to clean up. Irene reluctantly had to go back to work and diagnostic restaging exams. It went against her grain to leave me with a mess. I took her to the airport. I cleaned up with the rest of the neighbors. I had roof damage and fallen drywall from the first-story ceiling. The pool screen was gone—just six inches of twisted metal stuck out of the ground where each support had been. I took video and started to think about my insurance coverage.

After the cleanup and insurance negotiations, I flew back to Philadelphia to be with Irene during the upcoming scans and restaging procedures. I soon returned to Florida. In early September, another hurricane was on its way. I was using a lot of my air miles.

Charley wasn't enough! Labor Day brought Frances. We had days and days of rain. Frances was very slow moving. She hung around for several days. I was without electricity for a week. Irene called every hour on the hour, just about. I cleaned up, talked again to the insurance company, and went back to Philadelphia in a weakened state by mid-September. I didn't want to be away from Irene for long. I had been to every appointment and hospital stay from the beginning.

Now, I was watching the Weather Channel. Every Floridian was watching that channel now, no matter where they were in the world. Still another one was coming—another female. I flew to Florida again. Irene wanted to come with me. That was out of the question.

September 25, 2004, Jeanne looked like it was going to miss Florida. No luck. She made a turnabout and came right across our area, outside Orlando. We got hit again. I cleaned up and talked to the insurance company—again—and then I went back to our home in Fox Chase, exhausted, and fell into my smiling Irene's welcoming arms.

"God, I'm glad to be back with you, beautiful."

"I love you. It's good to have you here safely beside me, Tommy."

She said "Tommy."

Every now and then, Irene called me Tommy, which is what my family called me. She would imitate them with a smile. She liked it, but she wanted to distinguish me from my son, whom she always called Tommy, as I usually do.

After being hurricane-free for seventy-five years, Central Florida got hit with three of them in a six-week period. There was another near miss, Ivan. He didn't miss by far but a miss is as good as a hundred miles—still plenty of rain. We haven't had any since at our location.

Nevertheless, we still preferred Central Florida over any other part of the Sunshine State or Philadelphia. South Florida, the Florida coasts, and the northern Gulf states are threatened by bad weather far more often than Central Florida. Freezing snow and ice endanger us old and medically challenged folks far more than occasional tropical heavy wind and rain.

At last, when we were both home in Philly, we kept the appointments for restaging scans and other diagnostic tests, such as blood work, to see how Irene's CEA count was doing. The doctors wanted to see pictures from our trips. Naturally, we were proud to show them. We could tell they were happy for us. Our team's pleasant attitude improved our own.

Remission?

You know what I think about the word remission. The latest scans detected no lesions in the colon and no lesion on the liver! MRI scans showed no hypermetabolic activity in either the colon or liver. However, no one was using that word remission. Why?

Wow! Are we done? We've been praying, and it seems to have helped. Irene wants to do back flips. So do I.

No, we were not done! It had only just begun. The doctors warned that Irene should continue chemo at some point. Her disease was systemic. The restaging scans were negative, but scans can't detect growth of every tiny cancer cell. It was safer to continue chemotherapy in the infusion room at the hospital. Irene agreed, despite the anticipated side effects. The team believed in the possibility of Irene's survival. They wanted her to live. They comforted us, but they didn't use the term remission. We knew the reason.

We learned a little bit more about the various diagnostic scans used to determine size and growth rates of tumors: CT scans (commonly referred to as CAT scans), MRI, and PET scans. Each scan measures solid nodes, or, in the case of the PET scan, the actual metabolic activity of cancer cells. The PET scan has the greatest ability to detect the smallest amount of cancer and is used less frequently, usually when the other scans don't show distinctive nodules in the case of a patient, like Irene, with ongoing treatment. It is much more expensive than the others, which aren't cheap either.

If the CAT and MRI are negative in previous chemo patients, the PET is used to see if there is any detectable cell growth activity going on. In short, the CAT and MRI take pictures and the PET measures the actual division or growth of cells, then displays the activity. It can detect much smaller disease than the other scans but none of the scans are perfect.

As time passed and after a variety of scans, Irene had some bad side effects with those full-strength doses from the external pump going directly into her liver. The painful rashes and pimples on her face, upper torso, and arms didn't respond well to all the prescribed ointments. It also caused two fissures in a very delicate area, the anal canal. There was tingling in her hands, diarrhea, and very sore mucous membranes in every area a human being has mucous membranes. Use your knowledge of anatomy to recognize how painful that may be several times a day on a daily basis, for weeks, accompanied by diarrhea. Even brushing her teeth was uncomfortable, yet Irene wanted to courageously continue chemo anyway.

The fissures in the most painful area, the anal canal, were discovered in an exploratory exam. It was yet another procedure that Irene had to endure. There always was the associated discomfort of injected air whenever an exam entailed inserting a probe into certain openings of a patient's body. It takes several long hours to get rid of the air.

Bouts of diarrhea were agonizing. Irene said it felt like cut glass, even after the application of the ointments. I would hear moans and at times, screams coming from the bathroom. It was painful for me to hear her. Salves and ointments didn't work. It might take another surgical procedure if it didn't resolve itself. Eventually, the fissures cleared up—thank God.

10/15/2004, Friday: The doctor removed the arterial pump. The lead that connected it to my liver stayed there inside my abdomen when the balloon was disconnected. It wasn't necessary to remove it.—I. S.

Doctors took her off the irinotecan arterial pump. It hurt too much and complicated treatment. Irinotecan would be used again in smaller doses and delivered through the normal infusion process, her port, rather than directly to the liver through the lead from the external pump. But it had been effective!

According to the reports I read, when the doctor sedated her in the operating room and surgically opened up the area in the upper right quadrant of her midsection to remove the connection, the surgeon encountered clumps of blood inside the area. That may have contributed to her discomfort. It took two visits to surgery to completely evacuate all the fluid that accumulated. The doctor placed a drain in the wound to allow blood to escape. It cleared within three days, and the doctor removed the external, funny-looking rubber tube he called a drain.

11/30/2004: Ultrasound of my abdomen revealed no blood or fluid accumulation related to the pump removal. Doctor wanted to make sure the problem was resolved.—I. S.

12/22/2004: Another ultrasound. Doctor wanted to make doubly sure the area didn't have any buildup since the last ultrasound and that it was clear and clean of any residual blood or excess fluid related to the arterial pump and its removal.—I. S.

Interestingly, the surgeon made this latest incision to remove the pump along the same scar as the original. He did that not only for aesthetic reasons but because it reduced the chance of adhesions and scar tissue that a separate incision might cause. The surgical report stated that he folded up the pump lead on itself and tucked it away under some layers of tissue. He then sewed it in securely. It wasn't going to go anywhere.

Irene was accumulating several foreign objects inside her body. But that was fine with her. She hardly felt them. She never complained about them. That particular pump lead showed up on subsequent scans for years. Scan technicians would ask, "What's that?" I'd explain.

We had another treatment break for the holidays. Irene prepared a great meal. My sons, with different dates this time, loved Irene's cooking and Maria's supporting role. They loved Irene and Maria, too. Maria held them spellbound with the stories of her earlier life's experiences in the Ukraine and Germany and her nasty bosses at the sweat mill, where she worked for several decades since she arrived in Philly in 1951.

She told of the family's sea sickness on the troop ship that brought her, her husband and her children to the States. Who couldn't love Maria? Maria loved the attention. Irene sat smiling at it all and listened, delighted that her mother was happy and enjoying herself. All could see that Maria was happy telling her tales. Both Irene and I reflected on our own lives. It was peaceful and fun.

"Merry Christmas, Tom."

"Same to you, honey. Come over here under the mistletoe where I can give you a big hug and kiss."

"Why do I have to come over there? You don't need any mistletoe! You come over here by the sink."

"I'm on my way, sugar!"

We exchanged gifts on Christmas. We really enjoyed our second holiday season in our Fox Chase home. We frolicked a little but stayed at home most of the time. We treasured the control of Irene's condition, took Maria to mass, and prayed on Christmas Day. We settled back and waited for the arrival of the New Year 2005. Irene still wanted to accrue more and more leave time.

We often went out to dinner during our time off from chemo and surgeries. Irene would reach for my hands, and I'd slide mine across the table. Irene was still feeling subnormal, but holding hands comforted her. It widened her smile.

She'd been diagnosed with fourth-stage colon cancer; endured serious surgeries with the related hospital stays; threw two serious blood clots; wore an external pump that fed chemicals directly into her liver; faced numerous diagnostic tests and scans, all requiring bad-tasting drinks of contrast and two-hour waits lying on her back after being injected with dye or other contrast; and many, many chemo sessions during the past year and a half. Not to mention being exposed to a ferocious hurricane named Charley. Could anything else happen to her? I'm sorry to report that, yes, more bad news from the latest PET scan was looming over us. It was a good thing we took advantage of the time off and mixed in our mini-vacations.

Bad News: Back to the Infusion Room

03/21/2005: PET scan (most accurate type of scan) from my skull to mid-thighs. A few new small lesions on liver, spleen, right lower lung, and abdominal lymph node. Very disappointing.—I. S.

New lesions! Fox Chase doctors restarted chemo using irinotecan in reduced doses. It was effective in the past when combined with those two other drugs that make up the rest of the new cocktail: bevacizumab (brand name Avastin) and cetuximab (brand name Erbitux).

Irene's reaction to oxaliplatin, one of the first drugs infused, put her into too much distress, causing a delay in necessary treatment, so dosage had to be reduced during that earlier period. This time, doctors continued reduced irinotecan and those couple of others.

As I wrote earlier, bevacizumab (Avastin) was approved by the FDA for treatment in colon cancer chemotherapy in the United States some time in 2004, but it was controversial for a little while. Fox Chase got the authority to use it in time for Irene's restart of infusions. It's almost as if the FDA had Irene in mind. It paid to go for quantity. A relatively newly approved drug was approved just for Irene!

Another benefit of Avastin was it helped slow the growth of new blood vessels trying to replace damaged ones. That can be a problem in cancer patients, especially if they have a Greenfield implanted. Its approval was timely for Irene in treating her cancer but not in time to prevent the problem Irene developed with her Greenfield filter, which I previously described. Avastin wasn't available at that time, so it didn't have a chance to work to prevent those extra vascular growths in Irene's groin. It normally would have helped prevent them.

Avastin was initially approved for breast cancer, but that specific approval was later revoked by the FDA. That removal from the market caused quite a stir among the various breast cancer support groups, you may remember. A doctor may prescribe it in some cases, but insurance companies may not pay for it.

Cetuximab (Erbitux) is used in head and neck cancer but also in some forms of colorectal cancer. It has decent results. Cancer cells divide uncontrollably, which is the problem. Erbitux turns off the signal that tells those cells to divide, therefore inhibiting their growth. Irene's cancer cells had to be studied to determine if her cancer cells were the type on which Erbitux had the desired effect. They were.

To explain, there is a peculiar measurement used in colorectal and other cancer cases. It is a protein called KRAS. The acronym stands for *K*irsten *RA*t *S*arcoma. It is also a protein in humans. In 2009, the FDA updated how the effectiveness of certain drugs used in colorectal cancers should be labeled. Cetuximab (Erbitux) was one of those drugs. They didn't have this KRAS measurement back in 2005, but as it turned out, Erbitux was a good choice for treatment of Irene's cancer at the time.

Briefly, a *normal* KRAS is necessary to tell *all* cells how and when to mutate. It is basically an on/off switch. The messages can be slow, fast, or wild. This KRAS also sends the same signals to cancer cells. It's helpful for the medical team to know KRAS types in colorectal cancers. For what it is worth, Irene's KRAS was usually identified as the "wild" type. The wild type is the normal type. Its significance is that cetuximab (Erbitux) has a pretty good effect (59 percent) in patients with colorectal cancer and wild-type KRAS. The various KRAS types help medical teams determine the most beneficial cocktails to use, depending on the specific cancer involved.

Erbitux was working. Fortuitously, it had been the right choice for the team to use in Irene's treatment.

Erbitux can cause very severe itching and a rash, even pustules, all over the body. We sat beside a man during a couple sessions who had boils all over. He complained of not being able to sleep because the sores were so painful, especially on his scalp. He was in a miserable condition. He thought of just giving up. It didn't deter Irene. She did develop a rash all over her body, including her face, but even though it was hurtful and dreadful in many ways, she put up with it, and it resolved in a couple weeks. Ointments and salves were prescribed for the condition. I sadly watched Irene go through that phase. I was helpless, except to apply salves. I thanked God when she cleared up.

In addition, side effects, like shortness of breath, when Erbitux is administered can mean an allergic reaction. Nausea is a common side effect in many patients also.

The names of all these chemo drugs can get confusing. Some nurses use the brand name and some use the pharmacological name. I was taking notes during this time. We wanted to do exactly as the medical team dictated. We wanted to get it right.

We continued weekly chemo sessions with an occasional treatment break. I was at Irene's side every time, and I watched her eyes get heavy and then close. The cocktail would usually include a relaxant. I was grateful for the sleep and peace it brought to her. She looked happy because of that smile. In better times, that smile used to reach to the corner of her eyes, causing them to wrinkle a bit—the famous Irish smiling eyes, even though Irene was Ukrainian. My Irish must have been rubbing off on her.

When she slept, I noticed her smile was a little less pronounced but still discernible. I was so glad to be able to watch her as she grabbed a few winks early in the sessions. As the infusions went into the second, third, fourth, and fifth hours, however, they were often very uncomfortable for her. I was there with Irene every time.

Irene was super-human. During this period, she normally drove to work the next day without complaining. She anticipated needing to accrue leave time. She wanted to accumulate as much as she could. Not ready to retire again, Irene wanted to work.

We escaped a couple more times when we coordinated a vacation day with Irene's regular days off. Southeastern Pennsylvania vineyards also offer tastings. In addition to the wineries, Brandywine and Chaddsford are very historic. Sometimes we would just start driving and get lost, wandering through the beautiful scenery in Pennsylvania, our native state. We took advantage whenever we had the time. The doctors always agreed to skip a weekly session now and then to take a treatment break.

Sometimes we flew to Florida for a long weekend to see my family in Orlando and then drive over to her family in Bradenton. Life seemed normal for a while. Her family ran a small air conditioning business in Bradenton. Things were going pretty well for them. It was 2004–05, and the recession hadn't hit yet. There would be tough times ahead.

My family was doing fine at the time. Difficult times for them lay ahead also. Later, trouble hit when my niece, Kathy—the one who gave us the introduction to the director at Fox Chase—developed melanoma on her instep. She beat it, but a large scar tells the tale of her surgical experience. Her brother had a bout with cancer too. So did my brother. My father struggled with cancer in the '80s before he passed away in '85. I had cancer in 1990, as I mentioned. My sister survived cancer in 1997. There was no lymph involvement in any of these cases, fortunately. It still seemed like an epidemic among my clan.

Later, however, one of Irene's nieces, her brother's daughter, who lived in Pennsylvania, was afflicted with a double dose of cancer, breast and blood. She did not survive. I only met her a couple times. Once was on the campus of Fox Chase. She received treatment there also. She was a very pleasant, smiling woman who was working full time and going to school, pursuing her degrees. Cancer isn't particular about who it strikes.

Ironically, a heart scan during 2005 showed a perfect zero for calcium or plaque deposits in Irene's heart. Irene didn't know whether to feel good or not over that news. Neither did I.

In response to questions, Irene would often say,

"I'm healthy as a horse, except for this cancer thing."

If it hadn't been for "this cancer thing," she could have lived to be a hundred. Her mother is going strong, physically, at eighty-nine today.

As far as my health goes, my biggest medical problems are gastro-intestinal. Any other conditions are controlled by medications. My cardiologist once told me that I wouldn't die of a heart attack. Something else would kill me before my heart gave out, maybe a speeding truck or train.

My heart scan was very near zero. My brother, Michael, and I had the exact same tiny amount of calcium in the exact same spot. We also had very similar police careers. He has four published law enforcement fiction novels and another available this year, in 2013. I have a long way to go to catch up to him.

His latest published novel, *Imperfect Contrition,* is available as an e-book, too. The book is dedicated to Irene and Mike's brother-in-law who passed away two months before Irene. In it, Mike pays tribute to Irene. He created a new character named Detective Irene Stasurak. The character is newly assigned to Homicide Division in the story. He wrote it prior to Irene's death. He wanted it to be a surprise to elicit that great smile and wide eyes. He and I both wish the publishing process had gone quicker so she could have vicariously experienced her promotion to detective. I hope my brother's readers see more of Detective Irene Stasurak in his future thrillers.

If interested, you can search "InfinityPublishing.com" and then click on the "bookstore" button on the top ribbon; next, click the drop-down button to select "author"; finally, fill in "Cooney." All four books will be displayed, including a brief biography. His books are also on buybooksontheweb.com (BBOTW.com), Amazon.com, Barnes and Noble, and other sources.

Loyalty and Support: the Men and Women in Blue

There's no way I can skip forward in this chapter or go onto the next before I write a few paragraphs concerning friends of Irene and me who are still active officers and commanders on the Philadelphia Police Department. As is evident, Irene always was aware of the medical time lost in trying to fulfill her responsibilities of being a law enforcement officer. It took great management of schedules and super-human effort, at times, for her to make it into work.

When Irene was ready for duty again, thanks to the affection of our brothers and sisters in blue, we were able to arrange a transfer out of uniform assignments and into plain clothes: the Civil Affairs Unit. She had the qualifications.

The Civil Affairs Unit covered the entire city. It was a group of officers, supervisors, and commanders in plain clothes, who were at hand in crowds of protesters. They had two main responsibilities: be on site in the event of any disturbance; and protect the protesters in case of any attempted violence against them. The leaders of organized community groups coordinated their demonstrations with the police department that helped get the required permits, established the safest routes, and informed them of the law to which their obedience was required.

Relationships between *most* community groups and the police often are very cordial. Police must protect the various groups' freedom of expression and their right to assemble. Leaders of these organizations very much desire a good relationship with the police. The Philadelphia Police Department is proud of its relationship with the multitude of such groups that want to exercise free-speech guarantees.

Dozens of protest marches within Philadelphia occur every year, and rarely is there any problem with the legally organized groups when they conduct their activities. A few on the margins sometimes cause trouble. Usually the formal groups are composed of nonviolent people. Of course, uniformed personnel are always on hand just in case.

Anyway, Irene's transfer was a huge benefit for her. It saved time. She could go directly to or from duty and to or from doctor's appointments and chemo sessions in plain clothes. I could be with her too. Being in uniform with weaponry in the infusion room might be uncomfortable for other patients and staff. While in plain clothes, however, Irene could drop off her weapon at home or safely conceal it. Mine, too.

Performing personal responsibilities while in uniform is problematic. A uniformed officer is obligated to take official action or respond in a professional manner whenever a citizen demands it or a situation presents itself to his or her view. Otherwise, the civilians may lodge complaints. They don't want to hear that the officer is going to a chemo session, doctor's appointment, or pharmacy. They demand action immediately. They are not satisfied with the officer, off duty but in uniform and without a radio, telling them to please call police emergency, 911. The citizenry can be very unsympathetic and demanding at times and very cooperative at other times.

There was another advantage in Irene's transfer. Organized demonstrations took place at various times of the day and evening. Irene's work hours, shifts, and days off could be coordinated to adapt, somewhat, to Irene's needs. Treatments were always during the day. As long as she put the required number of hours at work during a specific pay period, no time needed to be deducted from her accrued benefits. And if she required time off, adjustments could be made to deduct the least amount of time as possible in conjunction with her use of holidays, vacation, administrative leave days, and sick days.

Over the last couple of years of Irene's employment, a computer program specifically designed for employees who are in a medically challenging position could not have accomplished it better. Thanks to our brothers and sisters in blue.

The officers, supervisors, and commanders who made all that possible are among the department's finest. Their loyalty and friendship to Irene and me cannot be equaled. And their loyalty to the service of Philadelphians in being part of a large governmental organization did not suffer at all. In fact, their service was superior because it demonstrated the character of the individuals within that unit and the whole organization itself. Besides, Irene was great at communicating with the members and the leaders of those community groups. They loved her too. Who wouldn't, with that smile she always wore?

I simply had to write something about the Civil Affairs Unit. In my mind and Irene's and in our hearts, we believed the brother and sister officers, her supervisors, and commanders all contributed to the quality of Irene's life during those dark and trying days, but they also helped extend Irene's life. There is not a doubt in my mind or heart about that fact.

I heard from them when Irene passed, and they were all heartbroken. I heard from many of the coworkers who knew Irene and who were touched by her during her career and in subsequent years.

And I just heard Irene thanking all of them too.

"Thanks, Chief! Thanks, Inspector! Thanks, Captain! Thanks to all my friends. You all helped make my life last longer. Thank you for everything you did for me."

I heard her. Didn't you?

Chapter Five

Wedding Bells

The day after we received the latest bad news from the diagnostic scans, I proposed to Irene. We'd been together about three years and by this time, I was deeply in love with Irene. It was time.

04/01/2005: Irene Stasurak (I. S.) becomes Mrs. Irene Cooney—I. C.!

We tied the knot. Note that it was April Fool's Day. When I called around inviting people to the private ceremony in a judge's suite, they thought I was pulling their legs. I'd been single for so long—more than twenty years.

I'd thought about asking Irene to marry me for quite some time, but so many things demanded our attention. I wasn't consciously putting it off. The timing just wasn't right—not until that moonlit evening while I was sitting on the porch glider. I watched Irene as she returned from inside the house with two glasses of California wine. She handed me one of the wines and sat down beside me, with a soft smile on her face, even though yesterday had been a very bad day. That smile hid a life of heartache and disappointment. She might have been thinking, *I've found someone, but will Tom stay with me? Will he stay?*

On that very pleasant evening in late March 2005, as she cuddled beside me, I thought about Irene.

Here was a woman, just turned fifty-two a couple months earlier, who had uprooted herself several times for the people she loved—her mother and me. She'd lived in an unhappy marriage for twenty years. She'd had very large disappointments early in life, too. The existence she breathed up to this moment and the heavy burden she carried around on her shoulders would cause many others to give up, just simply succumb.

I thought about her past, her present, and her uncertain future, and my heart just went out to her. I've admitted to having a soft spot for Eastern European women, but this feeling I had for Irene was much deeper. Irene was very bravely fighting cancer and all its derivatives for almost two troubled years. It had to weigh heavily on each breath and every step she took. I wondered if Irene thought she might be alone in the future. Would others take care of her? She might be feeling like her mother felt at nineteen, when Maria knew the Nazis were coming into her village, rounding up woman and taking them and her away, or worse, leaving her alone and helpless!

Both Irene's parents were ripped away from their own families, the memory of which to them must be inwardly vivid. Irene's parents led a dreadful life until they came to America and even then, their lives demanded hard work in the foundries (her father) and factories (her mother) that were prevalent in the industrial sections of Philadelphia in the '50s. That sweat-drenched employment afforded subsistence, not much more, to many immigrant families. The determination to survive and ultimately to thrive are qualities that Irene inherited from her Ukrainian ethnicity.

Irene attended a public high school but did not finish. For several years, she served tables and cleaned houses with her mother. Later, she struggled to get her GED and proudly accomplished that goal. She knew an education was necessary.

Her experiences made her the generous, compassionate, and pleasant person into which she developed. I loved her for who she was and her complete unselfishness.

Irene, and her sister, Tammy, eventually opened a beauty salon. The rent and expenses were too much to overcome. It didn't work out. That adventure was yet another dream of Irene's that didn't come to fruition.

About ten years into Irene's first marriage, in 1990, the city advertised for police officers. Women were urged to apply. She just made it under the age limitation. She recognized a great opportunity to fulfill a dream. The pay was decent and steady. Security and stability held out strong arms to Irene, but she would have to do it without support. Police officer—this was the job she was hoping for.

The entrance exam was the first hurdle and then the background investigation, the polygraph, and the psychological tests. It wouldn't be easy—ask anyone who has applied for and then gone through the police academy of a major city.

Most of the recruits in her class were fifteen years younger than Irene. Besides the physical requirements and book study required, the culture was not always exactly inviting to women in 1990. She was a female in a culture that was still hanging on to its man's world. Irene smiled through any degradation thrown her way and met all the requirements for her diploma. Graduating from the academy gave her fifteen college credits at five major universities in the area. Her resume expanded.

Irene's personality and demeanor earned her the respect she deserved. Irene was determined. She enjoyed going for every goal set before her during training: the obstacle courses; physical defense; the firearms range; defensive and pursuit driving; arrest procedures; the federal, state, and city laws—all of it. Irene was awarded her diploma and badge and proudly displayed both. I still have her badge. It seemed to Irene that she had a chance to finally find a better life than she ever hoped for. Irene experienced disappointment so early in life, more than her share.

All during the academy training and for almost the next decade, things were not going so well in her marriage. After almost ten years on the police department, she wanted to better herself and earn the gold badge. Irene longed to be a detective.

The money was good, due to a lot of overtime—time and a half court appearances on days off. Irene had plenty of time. She preferred to be in court, making overtime, than at home. In her marriage, she already was largely contributing to support herself and her mother. But she needed to complete the plan she'd had for several years. She wanted a divorce so she could have a chance at a somewhat more normal life. Irene strived for that chance. Maybe she would have it, someday. She continued to hope. She always had hope. She filed for divorce and wished it would happen quickly. She wanted to start afresh.

Irene signed up for my classes, and she came into my life, briefly at first, in 1999. The divorce wouldn't be final for several more months.

After twenty years, Irene and her mother, who lived with her, just left the home she cared for and fixed up over the last few years. She gave up everything except what was in their suitcases. Sandy helped her salvage a few beautiful Ukrainian eggs. She took her mother and those couple of suitcases and trudged off into a new and unknown life. The house, the furniture, pictures, and appliances all stayed behind. All except the suitcases and those decorated eggs.

Irene and Maria moved from one tiny apartment to another in bleak Philly neighborhoods, where she could afford to occupy quickly. Tiny streets and second-floor apartments became their way of life for months. By then, with her police salary, Irene earned and saved enough to buy that little house on Lardner Street with the cemetery in the rear where her cats played and chased squirrels. She watched the contented cats enjoy themselves. She felt like her cats—free. Irene owned her own home with no living neighbors behind her. She reverently smiled when she commented to others regarding the cemetery and her "neighbors in the back."

Irene was happy and hopeful. At no time in her life did she ever feel as good. Her mother was happy too. And she had another project. She fixed up her house. She bought new furniture and appliances. She took a barber chair out of storage from the salon that her sister and she briefly owned and put it in the basement.

Irene signed up for my Advanced Detective Prep Course in 2001, and we became an item after an egg sandwich, a steak dinner, many hours interviewing her mother, and a date in Atlantic City arranged by her friend and previous coworker, Sandy.

Irene placed very high on the promotional list. She competed against a few thousand officers all trying to get promoted. That's no small feat. Irene had plenty of that rarity—common sense. She had an excellent chance of accomplishing her goal of becoming a detective. She would have made a good one; I can vouch for that.

And then Maria wanted to go to Florida to be near her other children. She was getting up there in age. She was about seventy-nine. I got that phone call that made my heart sink. They were heading south.

After six months in Florida retirement, Irene was reinstated on the police department, March 3, 2003. We bought a house in Fox Chase, not knowing of the future constant visitations to the cancer hospital in that nice neighborhood. When promotions were announced, her name was first on the list. She was going to be promoted!

Then the fiercest hurricane of all hit her. She was diagnosed with fourth-stage cancer. She might not be able to pass the required physical exam; the overtime hours might be too much and conflict with treatment schedules. Tears trickled down that beautifully smooth skin on her cheeks. How much more disappointment could Irene take? But many more hurdles would appear along Irene's journey in years to come. Irene experienced devastation often, more than anyone deserves.

Why did I propose to Irene? I was sensitive to all the ups and downs in Irene's life from the very beginning and beyond, more than anyone else. I reflected on the various frustrations Irene was facing as I looked into her eyes while we sat on our side porch on that moonlit evening in late March 2005. Even though some people had known her longer, I believe I knew her best. I wish everyone knew her as I knew her.

I sensed that Irene worried that I was going to leave her after she was diagnosed with cancer. I'd known Irene since 1999. We were an item for more than three years by 2005. I didn't know it, but we would have another seven years together. Leaving her never entered my mind, but her insecurity had to insert the idea into her frail comfort zone. Many of Irene's wishes had been dashed in the past. My heart was both heavy and sad. But I knew I loved this woman, and I wanted to take care of her and be with her. I'd never felt so comfortable.

While we sat there on the porch, with Dusty looking on, musing over the past couple years since she was diagnosed, I could sense again that she was afraid of the present and the future—like Maria was afraid in 1942. Fear always lurked just beneath the surface for most of her life, even though that fear didn't stop her from trying to achieve a goal. Irene wanted, as we all do, a confirmation of her value and her worth. I noticed it even through her delicate smile. I wanted to allay her fear. I wanted to be with Irene all the way. I wanted her to feel very, very secure through this entire, treacherous journey. I wanted to ensure her comfort and let her know she would not go through this ordeal alone.

Because of my own battle with cancer, I knew the emotional impact. I wanted to be with Irene for richer or for poorer, in sickness and in health, unto death do us part. And that's the way it was.

She said yes! Irene jumped up then collapsed into my lap and arms. I felt that burden she had been carrying for years fly off into the moonlight. A few tears flowed. Irene wept a bit, a combination of relief and joy, I imagine. I'd made her really happy and comfortable, secure, and in love. And that made *me* feel wonderful.

In years to follow, Shakespeare's Sonnet XXIX became the best way for me to express how I felt about Irene. I recited it to her often during our time together and during her final days. The heroic couplet, the final two lines of the total of fourteen, expresses the feelings I'm usually unable to express. The couplet traveled through my mind, but I didn't vocalize the lines this time:

For thy sweet love remember'd such wealth brings
That then I scorn to change my state with kings.

We slowly rocked for a while on the glider on the side porch in that magic moonlight and slept very soundly that night in each other's arms after a couple celebratory glasses of California red wine.

Next day, I decided to call a previous workmate of mine with whom I served at the police academy twenty-five years earlier. He was a judge. I wanted him to marry us. I called him, but he had army reserves the weekend we wanted to get married. He made a suggestion that Irene and I immediately agreed to.

"Tom, do it on Friday the following week, and we'll do the ceremony in my chambers. I'm free that whole day. Invite your family and some friends too."

I don't think any one of us realized that particular Friday was April 1. I don't think we noted the irony.

Irene and I got our license at City Hall and notified everyone. My brother was my best man. Family and friends, including some from the Civil Affairs Unit and other places where Irene was assigned were given a tour of the judge's suite after the ceremony. He was honored often by community and colleagues, so the trophies and commendations lined his walls. One particular souvenir was a ball and chain from a closed state prison. Of course, I posed with him while I held that ball and chain. I posed with Irene while we both held it too.

Later, we drove to Florida for our honeymoon. There was no problem getting away for the honeymoon. Johnny Mathis was always playing in the background on the car's CD player. Irene would tell me I had a great voice when I would do a duet with him. Not true, at all. She said it anyway. I loved the way she wanted to please me, even when I knew she was kidding. I hope I complimented her enough. If I didn't, I should have. On the way, we stopped at Charleston and Savannah for a day each. We liked stopping by those southern cities.

On one of those overnights, I "spoke in tongues." Both Irene and I, while sleeping, have spoken in tongues, as Irene tagged it. The first time Irene brought it to my attention was when we stayed overnight in Charleston. She told me I was mumbling something, and she tried hard to understand just what I was saying. Of course, I had no idea what I said, but we both had good, solid giggles about it. When Irene told me about it, she couldn't stop laughing. That escalated to both of us breaking out in chuckles. It was contagious.

About a year later, we both had the chance to giggle again. It was Irene this time who was speaking in tongues during the night. That was her first time but not her last.

Back in Florida, we also loved our home. We threw a neighborhood reception party down there shortly after the wedding. Our Florida friends and family, who were unable to fly north for the marriage ceremony on such short notice, showed up, and a grand time was had by all. We misted up at the love and genuine happiness people felt for us. We could detect it. Great gifts!

Much has changed in the lives of those attendees in the past seven years and in our own. I just spoke to a neighbor who was going through colon cancer herself at the same time Irene was. She is doing very nicely. Down the street lives a woman diagnosed with cancer; she had a "clear" period, but now it's back. My next-door neighbor died of a very aggressive breast cancer three years ago. Her husband passed away last year of a form of blood cancer. He was a golfing buddy. Another golfing friend had two open-heart surgeries. His wife and he just had a beer with me in my man/woman cave. But life does go on, doesn't it?

Another good friend, at the same time Irene was suffering, was also doing battle with a spot of melanoma on his back. We could commiserate. He had lymph gland involvement and underwent radical surgery under his right armpit, which to this day is a little limiting. He is right-handed. He self-injected with one of the same chemos as I did many years ago. The injection chemo had a worse effect on him than it did on me when I was self-injecting. Everyone's reaction is different.

Let me sum up why I asked Irene to marry me:

She was very attractive. She was very appealing to me—a knockout to me. She was my type, physically. Irene had no inordinate demands for "things." She made responsible decisions regarding her activities. She had a balanced approach to her physical and material world, the world external to herself. She was generous with her own resources.

I noticed very early that Irene loved her mother deeply and did not consider her to be a burden. Internally, in matters of the heart, I witnessed her care and love for other members of her family and my own. When I fell down the stairs, I felt her heart was full of love for me. She shed tears when speaking to family members of other patients while we were in hospital waiting rooms. She empathized and sympathized easily. She was more concerned about the self-esteem of others than she was about her own. She was proud of me, which is no small accomplishment. She held friends close to her heart too.

Later, when Irene was told by a friend that the friend's husband was sick and cancer threatened, Irene's eyes filled. I could see Irene had a huge heart, and it often overflowed. She was generous with her feelings and her heart.

I've mentioned her abundant common sense and her ability to cut to the chase when presented with diverse facts. She didn't just repeat what someone else told her when it came to her worldview; she formed her own rational opinions after deliberating through various components of, for example, an investigation. Irene was an interested listener. She developed that mental discipline through all the years of her life, slowly at first, and then it came naturally. She was generous with her listening and her patience.

Irene loved people, and she loved animals, in that order. She was very spiritual on a personal level. She felt attached to her Ukrainian roots, especially when we would visit the Orthodox church, an hour north of Orlando. She knew of their suffering and that of other cultures. She enjoyed people, and she loved being alive. History, the Bible, and other people's lives were fascinating to her. Always, her focus was external. Irene was a very well-rounded individual who would be very easy to get along with. And to me, her soul mate, she gave her all. She was most generous with me.

We were very compatible in body, heart, mind, and soul. That's why I asked Irene to marry me. Even though, without a doubt, we all know love is far more complicated. I think you get the idea. Can you blame me?

Wrapping Up 2005; Going into 2006

04/14/2005: Restarted irinotecan, Avastin, and Erbitux. Trying to reduce or eliminate nodules found in my liver, lung, spleen, and abdominal lymph nodes. There was a spot up near and just outside the vaginal apex. I just hope it never goes to my brain. My husband *is right here beside me, just like he promised.—I. Cooney!*

Irene continued infusions at Fox Chase CC. The side effects were more severe than usual. If the scans scheduled for September were good, we would ask for a treatment break. Until then, Irene was hanging in there but always fearful of the cancer metastasizing to her brain. She dreaded that possibility.

We couldn't do any traveling for the moment. Irene went to work every day, even though she was feeling bad all the time. She still sported her smile, so no one knew how much she suffered—except me.

09/03/2005: When compared to the scan in March, no evidence of disease on my liver, spleen, vaginal vault, or abdominal lymph nodes. PET scan shows a small nodule in my lower right lung. Chemo sessions are working. Whoopee! Ready to celebrate.—I. Cooney!

10/25/2005: Scan, when compared to scan last month, shows no change. Lung nodule did not increase in size. Less than 1 cm. Nothing else showing up. In a couple months, we will beg medical team for a break from chemo over the Christmas holidays.—I. C.

By October 2005, intermittent scans to get baselines on the effects of the chemo were good enough to take a break from the nausea, vomiting, the itching, and fatigue. After convincing the medical team to give us a treatment break through the holidays, we leaned back and relaxed for the next couple of months. We were still very aware and concerned about the lung nodule.

We thoroughly enjoyed the holidays. We took a quick trip to Florida to visit relatives on Christmas. We went to Disney World with my sister's family to see the amazing fireworks display. Irene was awestruck, as she always was, when seeing something she'd never witnessed before.

In spite of all that was happening, we had a nice and loving holiday season, Christmas and New Year's 2005–06. We were enjoying a romantic part of our time off too. Irene and I would brace for whatever was in store for us in 2006, good or bad. Warming ourselves beside the fireplace and peering out the sliding glass doors in the family room, we contemplated our future holiday season celebrations.

"Tom. How many more Christmas and New Year seasons do you think we'll have together?"

"All of them, honey. All of them."

"Thank you, sweetheart, for saying that. I really love you, Tom. Do you know how much I really love you?"

"I do, honey, I do. You prove it every day of your life."

We would have six more Christmases together.

2006 New Year: New Problems

We were back in Philly by very early January for a scheduled PET scan. The two months off from chemo enlivened Irene. She wasn't feeling deep side effects, but they always lingered.

01/06/2006: Compared to scan in October, lung nodule is slightly increased to 8mm. Still very small. Will take a chance and continue our treatment break until April. That will give us six months relief. I want it to last longer. I need it to last longer. Chemo has been at least partially effective, and surgery is an option at that time if the nodule gets bigger. It's worth the risk for a few more months of feeling normal. Will consider surgery if the next scan shows any growth in that lung tumor. Doctors agree that the rate of growth is slow. Not a significant risk in taking a break.—I. C.

The medical team went along with Irene's request for time off from chemo. They could see how much she needed it. They surmised that at the rate of growth and type of nodule, there was not a significant risk of a few months relief. In addition, Irene's blood work disclosed that she was somewhat rundown, physically and chemically. Emotionally, she was also getting a little depressed. She misted up now and then. On occasion, I saw little tears on the brink ready to overflow with the slightest provocation.

The doctor prescribed something to decrease the depression. They knew it was unusual for Irene to mention her discomfort. We looked forward to simply relaxing for the next several months. Maybe meds would help to uplift her.

04/12/2006: Compared to scan of 01/06/2006, the lung nodule shows a definite increase in size to 1.5cm x 1.1cm. There is also a 1cm nodule on my right adrenal gland which sits on top of my kidney.—I. C.

The break was great while it lasted. But we were devastated again! Irene wept easily during the last three years. Tears were always close to falling. She cried a bit when we got the dire news that the lung nodule had enlarged. What a letdown. It was such an emotional rollercoaster.

04/18/2006: I had another mammogram done. No suspicious activity. Spending my life at doctor appointments.—I. C.

04/24/2006: They did a needle biopsy of the tumor in my lung. Results confirmed that it matches the original cancer type that was in my colon. It went through the lymph system to get to my lung, same as it did to my liver.—I. C.

Now there was something else hanging over Irene's head. Would it ever go away? How much disappointment can she handle? I could see how down in the dumps she got when we got the latest scan results. We hoped the lung tumor at least had not enlarged. But she didn't let anyone else know what was going on. Everybody thought all was well in the Cooney households. It was torture for Irene to constantly live with this horrible disease inside her body. People with cancer might imagine they can feel the cells crawling around inside them, but the cells don't crawl around; they just multiply.

05/02/2006: Scan. Lung nodule still there. Nothing on the adrenal gland. Chemo restarted today. Two more chemo sessions planned to mid-June. Same cocktail (irinotecan, Avastin and Erbitux). Side effects back already.—I. C.

05/30/2006: Memorial Day weekend. Scan shows nodule in lung not responding well enough. Getting ready for lung surgery by our favorite surgeon. Planning surgery for June 28.—I. C.

Irene had a long way to go, and she would fight all the way. She would survive six more years. I thank God and the medical teams. It was six years later almost to the day, on May 25, 2012, when we were told that Irene had three to six months to live, and the doctors recommended hospice care at home. She passed away less than a month after that horrific news.

Irene dealt with the new diagnosis and overcame any tendency to withdraw, succumb, complain, or just give up. At all our appointments and contacts with others, from beginning to end, whenever she was told how good she looked by the medical team, relatives, or friends, she would always point to me, saying,

"It's Tom. Tom is why. He keeps me going. Most of all, he loves me, and I love him."

I would glow. I would blush. And I would feel like a million dollars. That's my Irene! That's why I married her!

I wish I could hear those loving words again. I would deal with her condition and support her for nine more years if she needed me, until the day I died. People need someone to live *for*. I did not want to outlive her or my sons.

Traveling South

In late spring 2006, on one occasion we took a flight for a few days to Florida. Both flying and driving were uncomfortable for Irene because she was getting infusions again, but that wasn't going to stop her. At that time, her mother would be fine for the short period we would be away.

Maria had always encouraged us in the past to go away for a few days. Our next-door neighbor in the Fox Chase house was an accomplished and very wonderful woman, and the two of them took care of each other whenever Irene and I would take a break. A nurse friend lived two doors away and socialized with us. She always looked in on Maria too. Irene's relatives, who lived in nearby Bucks County, would be available in case of any emergency. They had helped us move into the house. They knew the area. Maria was well cared for.

We combined a couple vacation days to Irene's regular days off, as usual. I had a second car in the garage in Florida so, at times, we would just drive aimlessly, listening to Johnny Mathis and the *Mormon Tabernacle Choir's Greatest Hits.* The Tabernacle Choir album was uplifting for us with selections such as "Climb Every Mountain" and "You'll Never Walk Alone," plus several others. I had a Joni James CD too. I liked Joni James; Irene didn't remember her.

Cocoa Beach and Melbourne Beach are just an hour's drive away. Cocoa is a surfer's haven. The college crowd flocks there. A short and very scenic drive down A1A takes you to Melbourne Beach, a more sedate place to watch aqua-colored surf. There's a great Irish pub there, Meg O'Malley's. We always stopped in there for a bite whenever we headed toward Melbourne. I would have a Guinness.

Once, we headed south and bypassed Miami. Miami is only three hours away. We needed to be in Key Largo, just another hour on the road. A dear friend of mine passed away, and Irene and I went to his funeral, and I gave a eulogy. Afterward, I went out on the boat he used to lobster from. His friends and shipmates were aboard, too. I went out catching lobsters with them once before, as a guest in the late 1990s. We spread his ashes. I visited Key West in the past with my son, Chris. But Irene and I, together, never made it that far, due to time constraints on the trip to Key Largo. She had to get back to chemo sessions and work in Philly, too.

Later, when we lived in Florida for good, St. Augustine gave us a chance to drink water from the original Fountain of Youth. Hope springs eternal, as they say! It doesn't taste nearly as good as mountain spring water. We leisurely motored around Florida, finding very out-of-the-way little vineyards and antique shops and tearooms. That's how we found the tearoom near Lake Alfred.

Here We Go Again: Lung Surgery

We made a big decision at that time. We would remove this lung tumor, and then Irene, Maria, and Dusty would retire to our place in Florida. Dusty was feeling the loss of two cat friends. He needed to retire too. A friend of mine in the real estate business, a retired cop, put our house up for sale and sold it in a few weeks, with settlement in early July.

06/20/2006: Made all arrangements for lung surgery with medical team and surgeon.—I. C.

06/28/2006: Surgery at Fox Chase Cancer Center for metastasis in lower right lung. Very successful for total removal of lesion. The risk we all took to extend the break for another four months was well worth it. The escape did me good and the surgery was very successful. Surgeon said he couldn't be happier with the outcome.—I. C.

The surgeon cleanly removed the nodule, placed the required drains, and stapled the incision. Irene couldn't wait. She couldn't wait to shed that Foley catheter and the monitoring leads. And that darned nasal-gastro tube taped to her nose, going into her stomach, was irritating, as usual. She was discharged in just five days.

We made the decision to have the surgery at Fox Chase CC in Philly, rather than waiting until we completed our move to Florida. We were very comfortable around the surgical suites at Fox Chase and knew many of the nurses and technicians. We felt at home there. Later, we felt the same about the team at Moffitt Cancer Center and Research Institute in Tampa. But for now, Irene wanted to get that growth out of her body. It had been there too long.

We said good-bye to our team members of the past three years, all of whom wished us the very best. They told us to keep fighting, that there was hope. The director wished us well and was happy that Irene accepted his recommendation that we continue treatment at Moffitt Cancer Center. Moffitt, too, has an even broader national reputation.

Irene beat a path to the police personnel office. She started the day-long process of retirement—for the second time. But this time was for real. In spite of everything Irene went through, I could see a real glow about her. All the nurses we met always admired Irene's skin. I could now see how it radiated. I wanted to keep it glowing.

Irene's official date of separation from the PPD was July 6, 2006, just long enough to accumulate another holiday—Independence Day. Long enough also to have the last three years count toward her new pension. A separated employee had to return and stay for at least three years to have that latest period applied to the new pension computation.

We had the calculator out—something else to give us worry. She made it, comfortably. Her pension would be for a combined sixteen years of service, approximately. The pension was not enough to live on if she'd been alone, but Maria and Irene finally felt even more secure with the three of us and Dusty living together. I was happy about that. Maria also lived with us in the Florida home. Again, she had her own bedroom and private unshared bathroom.

Irene could trade in her accrued hours for additional months of medical coverage too. She did so. She expended six months during her first retirement. She was able to add some time back on the four years, six months she had remaining by contract. She added more than four more months of full coverage. That additional time would be very important when we had to search for coverage when her police department insurance ran out. It gave us a little more leeway.

In the meantime, we lived in a nice home near family and friends. We would be getting treatment at one of the best cancer research hospitals in the country. I was on Medicare and had a supplemental policy. There were no worries for me except to pay my premiums and deductibles, and that wasn't a problem. I was in decent shape along those financial lines.

I already retired from my business in 2004 and wrapped it up by early 2005. I did that when I saw that we had to take advantage of any break in treatments in order to enjoy life as much as possible under these conditions overshadowing us. Neither my heart nor my mind was there in the business anyway. Even so, not many of my students or clients had any idea of what was going on in my life.

I ran the business for more than twenty years. I started it part-time, back in 1984, when I got divorced from my first wife. I incorporated the business in 1985. I worked it part-time until I retired from the police department in 1993 and full time after that. Since that time, I expanded it, fortunately. I finally reached a plateau in life, in 1993, when I had only one job for the first time in my adult life.

But I did have something else to devote full time to now that I didn't have the business anymore—taking care of Irene. We used to joke about Irene taking care of me in my old age, because I was fifteen years older than she was. It didn't quite work out that way. It was one of Irene's deepest regrets—not her own illness, but who would look after me—and her mother—if she passed away.

Relocation to Florida

We drove to Florida with Irene still stapled up. Nothing was going to stop us. We had a clean bill of health and were starting fresh. We were not going to drive straight through, even though we were eager. When we decided to move to Florida, we put Maria on a plane. She was picked up by her family. Along the way, Irene and I visited Savannah again. That's a great little city. I was doing duets with Johnny Mathis. Irene smiled as we held hands.

07/11/2006: We went to Moffitt. Met with our GI (gastro-intestinal) clinic doctors and nurses and I had staples removed by a physician's assistant. [She would be with us for the next six years.] *Seems like a great team. They had already absorbed most of my medical history sent by the Fox Chase team.—I. C.*

Irene started putting her personal touch on our home. We replaced the family room furniture and the old hurricane-damaged lanai furniture.

Irene was almost feeling normal. I loved seeing her that way. Maria would be along shortly.

07/21/2006: Doctor decided on my cocktail. Gave us choice: do chemo at Moffitt or around Orlando somewhere nearer to home.—I. C.

The cocktail could be mixed and administered in either location, at Moffitt or locally. The location of diagnosis and treatment is extremely important.

07/31/2006: Tom and I made the decision to drive the 1½ hour trip to Moffitt Cancer Center from Orlando for chemo, rather than get it locally. Biweekly chemotherapy was recommended.—I. C.

It was convenient to get chemo close by, but it didn't work out for us. In our opinion, the treatment at that facility resembled a production line. I thought the nurse had too many patients assigned to her, all lined up along one wall, and not enough pumps. Irene always had her own individual pump at Fox Chase CC, as did all the patients. Chemo must be administered under very exact flow rates, not by eyeballing and finger-adjusting a plastic wheel in the delivery line.

We were disappointed but happy that we knew, in our opinion, how chemo infusions should be administered. After just two sessions we changed our minds and decided to return to Moffitt. They were very happy to see us back. We were happy to be back. Moffitt was a well-known research facility. They had the latest treatments available. And they always provided very personal and professional attention. I don't know why we even considered going someplace else.

08/02/2006: Regular visit to see how things were going. Lung and liver closely watched. Small concern. Nothing definite. Continue maintenance infusion upstairs fourth floor. See doctor in October. Doctor ordered a scan for 10/30/2006.—I. C.

The team ordered another baseline scan to have an up-to-date starting point for Irene's treatment and its progress. Diagnostic testing, scans, and blood work were looking promising.

Is Chemo Working?

After several biweekly cycles of chemotherapy at Moffitt during the summer and into the fall of 2006, doctors performed diagnostic tests. We then had good news: no evidence of the disease was shown on the scans. Free again!

10/30/2006: Whoopee! Great news! No evidence of disease. Treatment break again. Time to enjoy. Whoopee! Happy Halloween! Maybe get a job.—I. C.

Was this the end of Irene's cancer? Had she beaten it? No! But it was great news. It picked up our spirits. Never give up! No more chemo for another three months, at least, when Irene would get scanned again. At that time, maybe we would get yet another three months, and then yet another, forever, maybe. We could dream, and we did.

At Moffitt Cancer Center, the infusion facilities were expansive. There were two opposing wings. Each had its own nursing station. Each wing had at least a dozen and a half lounge chairs and was separated into large three-walled open-ended spaces for two infusion lounge chairs apiece, each with its own swing-out small TV. Curtains, when necessary or desired, were pulled between each chair, allowing a little more privacy than Fox Chase CC.

The reclining lounge chairs were ten to twelve feet apart, providing plenty of work space for the nurses. Two visitors could sit close to their loved ones within that large private area during the actual lengthy infusions. In addition, each wing had at least two private rooms with beds, for those patients who were in worse condition—penthouses, as Irene called them at Fox Chase CC. Those patients could receive their chemo completely lying down in a hospital bed. As time went by, Irene would use those rooms on several occasions, including the very last time she would get chemo late in 2011.

There were refreshments and supplies (Dixie Cups, Jell-O and pudding, sodas, coffee, tea, warm blankets, pillows, etc.) in an area between the wings that the visitors could fetch for the patients. At Fox Chase, a patient could get any of those refreshments, but a nurse, often busy tending others, would have to be asked. Of course, the visitor could make a long trip to the cafeteria when it was open and get ice cream, coffee, or Jell-O to bring back to the patient (you know all about Irene, me and Jell-O). It was a little more convenient at Moffitt.

At Moffitt, there was a waiting area for patients and visitors, adjacent but separated from the infusion wings, which could comfortably seat fifty patients, friends, and relatives, waiting for infusion chairs to free up. There was a big TV, sofas, and easy chairs, coffee and juice dispensers, and an exit door to a fourth floor roof patio, providing a good view of the University of South Florida campus on which Moffitt was situated. Irene's sister and family stayed with us in that waiting area a few times. They lived about forty minutes south of the hospital.

So far, I have not described the diagnostic test procedures. Certain scans require prep, drinking what seems like vast amounts of foul-tasting "contrast." The procedure didn't differ between Fox Chase and Moffitt. But Moffitt had results the same day as the scan was taken. Moffitt had very modern computer equipment. It certainly saved us some travel time. At Fox Chase, there would be a two-day delay, requiring another visit. That was no problem, because we lived so close to Fox Chase CC.

As the years went by, whoever prepared the contrast decided to flavor it. It helped a little but the patient had to drink a large volume of it, at least a liter within an hour. That's no exaggeration. Other scans require continual intravenous flow of a contrast or a colored dye. Irene was subjected to countless numbers of these kinds of procedures. If a patient is claustrophobic, it can become scary when rolled back into a CT, MRI, or PET scanner. There's not much room between one's nose and the scanner.

It takes some courage to undergo those tests. Some people just can't do them. I have seen patients regurgitate while trying to down the contrast as prescribed. Radiology Unit staff gave the drink to patients in four large paper cups on a carry-out tray and told the patient to drink one of them every twenty minutes or so. Irene never got the last one down. Irene would usually cheat a little and make a trip to the ladies' room, as I'm sure others have done, to pour away one of the cups. Nausea, remember, is constant in chemo patients. The technicians who understood said, "That's fine; three is enough."

For results like we had this last time, however, any discomfort was well worth it. The surgeries, procedures, and chemo infusions had worked—

again! Irene was a marathon runner in the world of cancer sufferers. (It pays to never give up!) All those surgeries and chemo sessions over the past three years were worth it. The pain and discomfort, the nausea, vomiting, fatigue, the itching and rashes, the diarrhea, rabbit-fur hair, and everything else on the list of side effects—all worth it.

Footloose and Fancy-Free

Now that we were free again, we took advantage of the time, naturally. We covered most of central Florida. We familiarized ourselves further with what was now Irene's home state. The state has several wineries. We visited them and sampled what the Florida grape had to offer.

Our favorite Florida winery was in Clermont, about an hour away. That area reminded us of the hills in the lower Pocono Mountain Range just north of Philadelphia. It's one of the few areas in Florida that is not flat. The rolling landscape was a reminder in miniature of the mountain resorts in Pennsylvania. You would never be able to ski at Clermont, but the grape was good because of those slopes. It was a very peaceful, pretty scene up there: blue, green, and white, most of the time.

The east coast gave us Palm Beach, Jupiter, Singer Island, Ft. Lauderdale, Boca, and several other resort areas. They were full of the rich and famous parading around, probably not as worry-free as their smiling faces might indicate. Who knows? The wealthy get cancer, too.

On the west coast, where Irene's relatives live, there was Anna Maria Island, Fort Myers, Clearwater, Dunedin, and Sanibel, Captiva, and Marco Islands, all beautiful places to visit, especially off season, when you don't have to dodge as many bicyclists.

We enjoyed our taste of freedom—two retirees in Florida. We certainly weren't unique. We meandered around the state of Florida whenever the spirit moved us. It was a carefree time, sort of. We always had our pool, too, and our beautiful sunrises.

We visited Irene's family up north. We jumped on a flight to the Philly area. We stayed over at their place in Bucks County. They were a wonderful couple who produced three very nice sons. They helped us move into our Fox Chase twin a few years earlier.

We always found time when we were in Philly to see my brother and his family. We drove down to my brother's vacation home in North Wildwood, New Jersey, to have a daylong visit with him and his wife, Pat. Mike and Pat have a son, Mike. My sister's name is Pat. You can imagine our family conversations with all the Pats, Mikes, Toms, and later, two Irenes. The four of us had a very enjoyable dinner over in Cape May.

And then, there were my sons, Tommy and Chris. We always dined at a nice restaurant with them and their girlfriends. Irene and my two boys adored each other. A few years later, in 2010, Tommy, my elder son, would marry a wonderful woman. Guess what her name is? Irene! He knew she was the right one when he learned her name. I knew he couldn't go wrong in life. It did get a little confusing, though. At family gatherings, during storytelling, we all had to specify which Tom, which Irene, which Pat, which Mike, which Don. My sister, Pat, has a son named, Michael, too. Pat is married to Don, and they have a boy named Don, besides their son named Mike. Got it all straight? You're good if you do. We can never get it straight.

But we had a wonderful three-month break again between scans, during which time Irene was doing very well, and we made the best of it. But Irene had a strong work ethic. No matter what was going on with her cancer and its side effects, Irene kept busy. One of her first projects in 2006, when she moved full time to the Florida house, a two-story structure, was to repaint the exterior. The house had been hit with three hurricanes in 2004 and about nine years of Florida sunshine by that time. Irene just smiled at me and pointed to the garage.

"Tom, it's time. Get your work clothes on."

Again, rollers and brushes were her modus operandi. My sons described her as washing dishes with one hand, cleaning the refrigerator with the other, and sweeping the kitchen floor with one foot while she stood on the other.

During one of the breaks, she applied for and got a job with Home Depot (employee discounts, you know). She got the job during the early part of the three-month treatment break we had when diagnostic tests didn't reveal any disease. She had hope! I couldn't stop her.

I knew she wanted to do it. Irene told me she wanted to feel as though she was contributing to the household. I tried to convince her that the household didn't need it, because she already was contributing. It didn't matter. She wanted to be even more generous. The few dollars of her salary would be split up to buy little gifts for me, her mother, and my sons.

But after a month or so, a scheduled scan showed a growth. It led to more disappointment. She had to quit. That happened twice during breaks in treatment at different times during the early years when we were in Florida, after her retirement from the police force.

During yet another treatment break period, Irene got a job with the school board in our county. That was with the help of a good friend and neighbor, the one who had skin cancer on his back. That effort lasted only a few weeks, and she again had to quit. That was the last time she considered actually taking official employment. It was getting tougher to keep her chin up. But Irene never lost hope.

We were in good financial shape. Irene never had to work again, once she retired from the police force, and we would live very nicely. But Irene gained self-worth through her labor. She wanted to keep busy, too. Think about it. If you suspected you were going to die, and you were a hard worker your whole life but were unable to gain employment, what would be your options? Would you go on a world tour and complete a "bucket list"? You have treatment and chemos to get. You're not actually completely free to roam, unless you have given up hope for survival and forgo medical attention. And you may be nowhere near your family when you died. Bucket lists sound good for the movies, but most of us are not alone—we have caring families.

I'll tell you what Irene wanted to do. Across the street was my friend who fought melanoma. He and his wife had no children, but they had two wonderful golden retrievers. My friend and his wife were professionals. They spent a lot of time at work. They were very busy people. I let out their dogs on occasion, when my friends couldn't make it. We socialized together. We trusted each other. They loved Irene. But their home was not kept up the way they would like it. They saw Irene's disappointment when she had to leave the jobs she had acquired. They knew her habits around our house. So they described their situation and their need of regular house cleaning. Guess who volunteered to clean their house? Yes. That's right. My Irene!

Irene wanted to feel valuable to her neighbors. A couple times a month, Irene crossed the street and spent a few hours cleaning their home. Her mind floated back in time to when she and her mother scrubbed floors and bathrooms in order to supplement their income. Irene would come home elated, having performed a job well done. She always came home after her "job," exhilarated and smiling. Then she would relax in a nice bubble bath. We'd have a couple glasses of wine.

Irene was a superb housecleaner; no necessary house chore was beneath her. The couple across the street was totally surprised to see Irene's end product. It was dazzling.

However, all good things must come to an end. In Irene's case, it was usually more bad news, similar to what stopped her careers at the Philadelphia Police Department, Home Depot, and the Osceola County School Board.

Our friends across the street lost their great savior that rescued them from their busy schedules. Of course, they were both heartbroken—but for Irene, not for the loss of a maid service. Remember, he had suffered through melanoma, and his wife was right there with him through the entire terrible experience. They understood! Neither Irene nor I had to go into any long explanations. It wasn't necessary.

Further proof of Irene's work ethic and worldview during this period of our lives: she never wasted any time. It was so valuable to her. For several days, off and on, she got down on her hands and knees and cleaned the grout between the tiles on our floors. Most Florida homes have extensive tile work. Basements are rare so first floors are on slabs that easily support the weight of tiles: entrance hallways, bathrooms, and the work areas and eating areas in kitchens, for example. That's a lot of square footage. I tried to stop Irene from cleaning the grout, but my effort didn't work.

I'm lazy in my old age. Selfishly, I wanted her to just lounge around with me and travel when we could. But I understood what Irene was doing, and I was happy for her and supported her in doing whatever she wanted to do. If she wanted to go overseas or to the wine country again, we could do that too. Wherever she wanted to go, I was all in. If she wanted to dip her toes in seawater or do dishes, I was all in with Irene. We could afford to do whatever endeavor she wanted to undertake, thank God. All of Irene's activities gave Irene *value*. Nothing, not even cancer, was going to steal her self-worth from her.

Irene was always smiling, but she was struggling to live in her own way too! Cancer was her motivator. If she'd been an artist, she would have created a new canvas every day. If she'd been a dressmaker, she would have designed a new style daily. Irene and her mother cleaned houses in the distant past, so that was what she wanted to do.

Our emotional state was as expected, but we kept on the happy faces. People thought Irene's illness was all over, and we were back to normal, just like everyone else. "Boy, that was something, but you beat it," people would declare. That comment was not close to being true, but most people didn't know.

We knew, however, that the disease was in the lymph system, and there was always a chance it would show up somewhere at some point. And the doctors always reminded us that Irene's cancer was systemic. The medical team never gave up either, but they were cautious. They were striving for *quantity*. Irene and I wanted *quality* too. In a way, we were achieving both, Irene-style.

It's not a pleasant condition to face every day—to have it on your mind every hour, day and night. A similar situation would place many people into limbo or worse. The mental anguish was incessant. It was a constant problem that continually shaped our world view.

When we tried to make any plans, we had to take into consideration certain questions: how should we anticipate the future? Should we say "if" the cancer comes back? Or should we say "when" the cancer comes back? It didn't stop Irene, even though it was beginning to slow her down somewhat after three and a half years of it. Irene would sometimes wonder what the next day would bring let alone months or years in the future.

"Tom, I think this is going to be our lifestyle for the rest of our lives: cancer on, cancer off. Can you handle that? You won't leave me, will you?"

I knew how Irene was worrying about staying alive. She was also worrying about my health and something happening to me. I tried to comfort her when she was feeling low.

"Honey, please don't say that. I'm staying right here beside you. I'm here beside you until the very end—either my end or yours. Remember my vows, honey, remember my vows. Don't worry."

"God, I'm happy, Tom. I could not go through this without you."

"Thank you, sugar. But I'm no good at scrubbing floors, honey. They told me so when I was in the air force."

I had a grin on my face. Irene laughed. She came over to me with that broad smile. She put her arms around me and hugged me. Irene looked right into my eyes and told me, "I love you."

I blushed. I felt fulfilled. Irene stepped back from me a little but still was holding me. She shot a glance at me and implied a honey-do list. "So you're no good at scrubbing floors, according to the air force. What did they say about cleaning and balancing the chemicals in a swimming pool, Tom?"

"Uh. Nothing, Irene. We didn't have any swimming pools."

"I see a little tiny bit of algae in the spa, handsome."

"Okay. Okay, honey. I'll get to it first thing tomorrow morning!"

"I still love you, Tom. Don't worry."

Chapter Six

The Liver Again: Left Lobe This Time

01/2007: After a few months without chemotherapy, diagnostic tests showed a small lesion again, in the left lobe of the liver this time. Nothing in the lung after six months. The doctors are going to start chemo again to see if they can get rid of it or slow the growth.—I. C.

01/24/2007: Chemo restarted. Feeling bad. Threw up several times, very fatigued, chills, fever. Vomiting lasted three days. Dry heaves. Muscle and joint pain, diarrhea. Compazine didn't help. Stopped chemo.—I. C.

Besides not feeling well, Irene participated fully in agreeing to have surgery on the left lobe of her liver. The scans determined the node was near the surface and accessible so the surgeons were able to enter through an incision and "wedge" the tumor out of Irene's liver. They didn't have to remove the entire lobe. They removed most of the right lobe of the liver last time, remember.

In the meantime, we scheduled colonoscopies for February. We drove to the appointments together and had them, one after the other, in the same facility.

02/05/2007: Tom and I had colonoscopies performed in a gastroenterological clinic. Both of us were "no evidence of disease." We had scheduled them together after the holidays. Afterward, for several hours, the procedure causes a lot of expelling of the air they pump into you.—I. C.

02/07/2007: Scans after the chemo sessions revealed the liver lesion is growing (it's about an inch in diameter). We scheduled surgery. Our new oncologist requested my participation in a cancer tissue study for my upcoming surgery to remove the liver tumor and allow slides to be kept for future research. Of course, I agreed.—I. C.

02/07/2007: Same day our oncologist asked me to participate in another study—immunotherapy. It is sponsored by Duke University and National Cancer Institute. Study is to evaluate effectiveness of a drug in preventing recurrences in patients who had colon cancer that had spread to the liver, and then after a liver surgery there was no detectable malignancy for an extended period. Tom and I reviewed the info provided, and we decided to do it. I hope I qualify after my surgery.—I. C.

We met with the surgeon. She requested several diagnostic tests: PET scans, ultrasound, etc., so she completely mapped the area around Irene's liver and stomach. The surgeon was very professional and at the same time very nice. She smiled a lot too. We liked her. She explained she didn't anticipate any major problem. Irene's current health condition was acceptable to undergo the procedure.

We would see more of her in the future, and we developed a nice, friendly relationship, which is good to have with your surgeon. In her subsequent reports, the surgeon regularly described Irene as "a very pleasant and cooperative …female." That is a common description that most of Irene's doctors at Moffitt wrote in their reports. All the way through May 2012, including Irene's final clinical research trials, the professionals' reports described Irene as "a lovely Caucasian female," "delightful Caucasian female," "a cheerful Caucasian female," "a very cooperative Caucasian female," and similar flattering appraisals of Irene. Irene was so easy to get along with.

Everyone who met and knew her described her with endearing phrases. She was such an angel. Irene's personality wasn't lost on any of her caregivers. Her type is so rare.

02/11/2007: I was admitted to the very well-equipped hospital. Liver (wedge) surgery will be performed, as the lesion was near the surface of the left lobe of my liver and close to my stomach. No other lesions were detected in the liver. Scans showed all that conglomeration of veins around the Greenfield too.—I. C.

02/12/2007: While inside, doctor wedged the liver lesion, but she also removed some disease at my stomach exit area. She cut out all she saw there. Also a lymph node that was swollen and didn't look right—she got it when she was in there. Why not?—I. C.

Our very pleasant surgeon always explained the procedures to us, diagramming them with Magic Marker on the hospital room communications wallboard. When the surgeon cuts away an area, the best practice is to remove it beyond the edges of the spots observed. Her operation was video-assisted—very cutting-edge, if you'll forgive the pun. The examination of Irene's tissue postoperatively indicated the borders were negative for disease. That was good news. The surgeon got it all. We really had no idea that the cancer had metastasized to Irene's stomach region.

However, in cutting and then suturing that area, the exit of Irene's stomach near the first segment of the small intestine (duodenum) was necessarily kinked slightly. We had to keep an eye on whether or not it interfered with digestion when Irene was able to eat again. It was also known from previous scans that Irene had a small hernia near that position. It wasn't important to do anything about it just then. It was the least of our worries.

Later, in May 2008, when the hernia caused more pain than usual, they considered repairing the hernia but other issues intervened. The hernia remained for the rest of her life and even though it caused constant mild discomfort, it never caused any major difficulty.

The kinking was a more important issue. But four days after the operation, an upper GI study indicated no blockages or leaks. Irene was eating hospital food again. She was discharged six days after enduring the operation, that nasty NG tube again, and staples. She was glad to be home.

02/18/2007: Discharged. Whoopee! More scars on my tummy. Floor nurses all very friendly and professional. Still have pain. Dilaudid relieves it. Restricted diet for a while and no heavy lifting. Any fever, call them.—I. C.

02/28/2007: Follow-up visit. My stomach and duodenum area became slightly restricted but worth it to remove the disease. I was able to eat near normally within a short time after the surgery. Whoopee! Surgeon gave me a clean bill of health.—I. C.

Freedom! After Irene was home and fully recovered from her latest operation, we had some time to ourselves. We kept a few follow-up appointments at Moffitt, and all was going well. We scheduled baseline CAT scans for May, the mandatory waiting period to be free of disease for that immunotherapy study. We hoped the scan showed that Irene was clear of detectable cancer. We didn't do any long-distance traveling. We just enjoyed our freedom as much as possible while anticipating the scans and their results.

I did any doctoring I needed to do and may have even played a round of golf. I really don't remember the last time I played a round of golf.

We took Maria to mass at our parish, St. Thomas Aquinas Catholic Church. Thomas is my patron saint. We also found a Ukrainian Catholic Church about an hour's drive north. We attended mass and other functions at the small church a few times. Maria was right at home with all the Ukrainian speakers who attended. The dialect of the younger immigrants was quite different from the seniors, Maria noted. It had a very definite Russian influence, according to the annoyed elders, resulting from Moscow's influence and oppressive control of the schools during the Soviet era. The pastry treats they had after ceremonies were very tasty. I still get occasional pieces of mail from the pastor.

05/01/2007: Restaging scans. Surgeon did a very good job in getting out all the nodes. I'm clear. That means I can be eligible for the immunotherapy study. Whoopee!—I. C.

Immunotherapy: Potential Deliverance?

05/09/2007 and 05/21/2007: Scans to assess my eligibility. These were required by sponsors of the immunotherapy study and to map my insides. I qualify. If it is effective for me, it may be a grand slam home run. Trial drug hopes to keep cancer from returning. Whoopee!—I. C.

Irene eagerly participated in the immunotherapy program. Basically, immunotherapy attempts to "train" the immune system to shrink or eliminate tumors. It aims to extend a person's life (quantity) by stopping the growth and spread of the disease.

In Irene's case, there was a procedure called leukapheresis in which a catheter was placed in her femoral artery, and Irene's entire blood system was recirculated again and again, collecting certain types of blood cells. It continued hour after hour so that a sufficient volume of specific cells was collected. It took all her strength.

The reports stated that she handled it satisfactorily, but I know what the involvement did to her over the course of several days. Irene's view was that it could have a very positive result—possible greatly extending her life expectancy, maybe even complete freedom from disease. She was always optimistic but said she hoped she never had to go through that procedure again.

You might remember my explaining the time when Irene got a catheter, and the physician's assistant inserted it in the right femoral artery after I told him it would be better if he used the left side. I explained to him about the Greenfield filter causing many congested blood vessels in the right groin area. Well, *this* was that procedure, which caused Irene to scream and me to scream at the PA.

The mechanical process of leukapheresis is not unlike dialysis in principle, but it filters blood cells not waste products. Those collected blood cells were shipped to a lab, and a serum was custom-made based on Irene's specific cell construction. Then that serum was returned to Moffitt for injecting Irene every twenty-eight days for four months. In order to participate, a person had to be clear of detectable disease after a liver resection for metastatic colon cancer.

In this immunotherapy study, there were seventy-two patients from around the United States, twelve of whom were from Moffitt, including Irene. She was fortunately breathing rare air at the time, considering all she experienced so far in four years following a fourth-stage diagnosis. The participants were randomly placed into one of two groups. One group received a placebo, and the other received the study drug. It is not common to use a placebo, but if one is used, the administrators let the patients know a placebo is part of the study but not who receives it. A patient never discovers in which particular group she is placed.

After several regular visits for blood work, Irene had a physical exam to see how she was feeling and responding to the relative freedom that the study provided. Irene did not receive any infusions during the four months of the study. We were relatively unburdened again. She remained cheerful and optimistic during that period, all the time worrying on the inside. She wasn't job-hunting anymore, either.

09/18/2007: I finished my first couple rounds of injections over the last twenty-eight days. Causes burning sensation down my leg when injected. It's a lot easier than chemo. I'll be starting again and be done in November.—I. C.

11/19/2007: Follow-up visit. Finished study. I feel very good. Just some diarrhea and joint pain. Blood work good, too. Maybe it's working. I will have restaging scans and blood work every three months. Doctor encouraged me to continue annual mammograms. Might be time for a trip overseas.—I. C.

The year-end holiday season rolled through without incident. We were very thankful that Irene was feeling okay. The constant fatigue, however, really never left. We took Maria to Bradenton on both Thanksgiving and Christmas, with Johnny Mathis Christmas carols in the background—and a reflected image of a cross on a metallic-domed building halfway down Interstate 4. The vision followed us as we drove by at 75 mph. We looked for it every time we traveled in either direction between Bradenton, Moffitt, and home. It was both eerie and uplifting. Is it spiritual messaging? We always hoped it was.

On another of our favorite albums, Johnny sang his rendition of "Maria" from *West Side Story*. I would sing a bar or two and look into Maria's eyes. What the devil was wrong with me? I never did that to my own mother; too self-centered at the time, I guess. Too busy! Too young!

Maria lit up and an unrestrained smile spread across her face. Sometimes, I was saddened at that smile, with her missing and worn teeth. It was stark evidence of a deprived period during her formative years. Maria's youth and early adulthood were not as plentiful as she would have preferred. How can anyone, knowing her story, not simply adore Maria? She and I always kissed lightly on the lips when we greeted or parted. It was never a simple hug or hurried peck on the cheek. She wouldn't think of that pretentious, pursed-lips "air" kiss you see a celebrity throw at someone across the room.

At her sister Tammy's home, Irene always helped with the cooking and cleaning up, as usual, no matter how bad she felt. We managed to stop by my sister's later on Thanksgiving Day, while on our way back from Bradenton, trying to see everyone on the same day. We enjoyed our second Thanksgiving dinner.

01/25/2008: Regular visit. Will continue maintenance 5-FU. Not feeling well. Usual stuff. Will have scans in about three weeks. Will know more then. I'm getting severe headaches, and I can't stop grinding my teeth. Nervous.—I. C.

Yet Another Setback

02/19/2008: I must have been in the placebo group. Cancer is back. Several liver lesions. Nowhere else, though, if that is any consolation. Another big disappointment. High-dose something called capcitabine (Xeloda), plus Avastin. Sounds like my old nemesis oxaliplatin might be involved, too. CAPOX plus Avastin.—I. C.

As you can tell by the acronym in Irene's note above, CAPOX, the newest cocktail, includes oxaliplatin. Irene rescheduled biweekly chemo infusions after the immunotherapy program failed in her case. We did sincerely hope it helped others.

A weak ray of hope dangled, but it was not low-hanging fruit. We were told there was a slim possibility of what the doctor called a "rescue surgery" on Irene's liver node, as long as the lesion that developed didn't spread to other organs in the meantime.

02/25/2008: Bad reaction to newest cocktail. Darned oxaliplatin.—I. C.

02/27/2008: Restarted chemo again. They'll try oxaliplatin again (reduced dose), along with the Xeloda and Avastin.—I. C.

Our oncologist was moving to Texas—his last day with us was March 14, 2008. He accepted an offer to rise in the ranks of oncology at M. D.

Anderson Cancer Research Hospital, which is one of the best in the country. We wished him well and expressed our gratitude.

03/18/2008: Scheduled for another round of CAPOX infusion, but it was held off. They put me right into the hospital. I was admitted to Moffitt Hospital dehydrated. I have had severe diarrhea for the last several days. Received fluids to hydrate me. Diarrhea probably due to CAPOX, according to doctor. That oxaliplatin is effective but doesn't agree with me.—I. C.

03/19/2008: Scan compared to last one showed four new lesions. Biggest is about 1½" x ½" plus enlarged lymph nodes in area. Talked to doctor about repairing my hernia (it's looped but not obstructive). I have a lot of pain in my midsection; maybe it's the hernia. Could be cancer, too.—I. C.

Irene was discharged after this latest hospitalization but not before a couple days of hydration and medication. The diarrhea that got her admitted stopped with regular doses of meds while in the hospital. She was told to continue the meds at home. If the problem returned, she was to call Direct Referral Center and arrange to be admitted again. We didn't have to go back. The diarrhea mostly resolved with the medications at home.

Irene's biweekly chemotherapy continued through the next month when the new oncologist would decide what to do.

We met our new attending oncologist while Irene was in the hospital for hydration and diarrhea control, so we set up our next appointment with him for April. A baseline CAT scan would determine if there was any improvement or regression.

We discussed available options. He reminded us that oxaliplatin was stopped, not because it was ineffective—it worked well on Irene's cancer—but because of Irene's side effects from it. Irene, brave spirit that she was, agreed to restart chemo with the oxaliplatin combination in the face of all the side effects she knew she would endure. The infusions were in the safest place possible. All her attending medical personnel hovered around her. She wanted the cancer out of her body. She was ready to do anything and suffer anything. I supported her. She wanted to live. She would do whatever it took. Courageous woman!

04/15/2008: I told the team I had severe, watery, whitish diarrhea over the last several days. Fatigue, nausea, dehydration. I'm still grinding my teeth; my jaw and face are sore. I have sores in my mouth. I have headaches. My feet and hands are red and painful. I feel miserable. They said acupuncture may help headaches. I prefer chiropractor for my headaches.—I. C.

I saw that Irene was beginning to tire, but she remained resolved to win this battle. She had many of the side effects on that long list I created earlier in the book, plus jaw and face pain, probably from the chemo, according to the doctor. Her hands were painful too. She felt pretty low, but she refused psychiatric referral when offered. She just wanted something for the migraine headaches and the depression. The doctor gave her the prescriptions. I thought a trip might do us both good when she felt better.

05/13/2008: Switched to a lower dose of oxaliplatin. In the interim, since last month, diarrhea was too severe. Tension headaches continue. Switched back to another old reliable, FOLFIRI.—I. C.

We were still thinking about asking to put off a scheduled chemo for just a few days. We could use a vacation from it all—maybe to Niagara Falls this time. Unfortunately, Irene wasn't up to it, but we put off a chemo infusion for one week anyway. We needed a break. We just stayed at home and tried to relax in between chemo sessions.

06/17/2008: Still doing chemo every two weeks. Feeling a little better with irinotecan. Something new; I'll go home with a portable again but it's hooked to my port, not my liver. It's 5-FU.—I. C.

The portable bag infused precisely over forty-six hours—not forty-eight, mind you. A home health nurse came to our home to disconnect the lead coming from her port after the forty-six hours and then flushed the port. The nurse also took blood samples for labs at each visit. This happened every two weeks after regularly scheduled chemo sessions at Moffitt Cancer Center. They arranged for us to receive associated supplies, too, for the nurse's use. Supplies included bandages, port leads, and flushing and blood-thinner syringes.

Irene and I made the trip to Moffitt many times that summer of 2008. She had chemo during June, July, August, and into September for her regularly scheduled infusions every two weeks. Every month or so, we pushed a session back a week and took a break. The doctors saw no problem with our improvised scheduling. The pace we set seemed to be working for Irene. She began to brighten and appear more enthusiastic. She really needed those occasional breaks.

07/16/2008: Good news. Irinotecan, 5-FU, and Avastin having an effect. Nodules slightly smaller. Still have hand and feet pain, jaw hurts, nausea, and that darn fatigue. Gave us our freedom until September. Heading to West Coast in a couple weeks. Then, Tom's oldest son and girlfriend coming down a few weeks after. She is really nice. Her name is Irene.—I. C.

I was thinking that we didn't enjoy our pool enough lately. It was a hot summer day and floating around on a raft sounding like a good idea to me.

"Honey, let's get into the pool for a little bit."

We changed into our bathing suits and gathered some towels.

"You have great legs, Tom."

"You probably tell all the guys that, honey. I'll get a couple glasses and then we can have a dip."

"Do we have any Beringer, Tom?"

"Yes, we have the Zinfandel blush you like. And there's still a little left in that bottle of Cabby. I'll finish that up."

"Sounds like a plan, Tom. Thank you."

California Wine Country—Again

Napa Valley was great, but we hadn't toured Sonoma or stood in the middle of the redwoods up there in northern California and lower Oregon. Irene didn't need to worry about getting back to Philly to resume her duties as a police officer this time. She was retired. And I didn't have any contracts or seminars to get back to.

This time we flew to San Jose, California. We wanted to take the tour of Alcatraz and see Al Capone's jail cell, along with the lairs of other famous convicts from that gangster-busting era, so we drove down to San Francisco. We pre-purchased the tickets so we were assured of boarding the ferry to the island. We drove to the dock, boarded, and went to the open deck topside. It was a very cool and windy day. On the island, we wore headsets, and a narrator's voice followed the route in the dilapidated building that the guide led us through. We saw the Chicago mobster's cell and several others. Each of us had our picture taken in Scarface's old homestead.

There was one jail break that no one is sure about; that is, its success or failure. Three very creative inmates, two of them brothers as I recall, rigged a makeshift inflatable raft and pushed off the island during a bleak night. They never surfaced again; that is, they were never captured. Forgive the pun; I can't help myself.

As interesting as Alcatraz was, our prime destination was Sonoma Valley. Neither one of us had ever been there. Again, we stayed at a gorgeous little B&B with a beautiful garden. A bottle of wine was in our room when we entered. That was better than a chocolate mint.

Sonoma Valley is not as well known as Napa Valley, but it is gradually becoming a more popular area. More and more coordination in the public relations effort on the part of the wineries is increasing tourism. Sonoma is quainter than Napa, with not as many expansive vineyards spread across the rolling landscape. But it was just what the doctor ordered—relatively quiet and very romantic. We needed that kind of atmosphere.

There was a retail winery there, and we joined a wine club. At this roadside winery, outdoor picnic tables were available under the trees. We sipped wine and ate slivers of every kind of cheese on earth. Before we left, we signed up for shipments of the featured wine of the month. The winery shipped them to us for several months until we stopped the membership. Neither we nor our families and friends could consume it all. In addition, an adult must be available to sign for the carton and we could never be certain we were home. It became an inconvenience trying to coordinate with Federal Express.

I mentioned earlier that our favorite winery was Beringer's. It is in Napa, the next valley over from Sonoma. A mountain pass meanders its way between the valleys, so we decided the drive might provide some great views. We were not quite sure where the road was or how difficult the venture might be, but we set off to find the pass anyway.

We were glad we did. As we drove up one side toward the highpoint, we knew the altitude because at every thousand feet, our elevation was painted across the macadam. Up and up we went. At the top, we paused, sucked in that great air, and took some pictures. The panorama was breathtaking to us Floridians. We were glad we'd taken the gamble. Understand that the mountains are not the snow-capped Rockies. I don't remember exactly, but the highest altitude was probably four thousand to five thousand feet above sea level. We still enjoyed the great view, though.

Down we went, and we didn't stop until we got to Beringer's. After a little bit more tasting and cheese, we went back to our B&B via the same pass connecting the two valleys. We wanted to get a good night's sleep and then drive northward to one of the nearest redwood forests on the morrow.

Redwoods, or Sequoia trees, are huge. There's not much sunlight penetrating the paths tourists walk, so the pictures we took are pretty dark. Plenty of miles-long walking trails meander throughout, but Irene and I had our physical limitations. We just took in the majesty of the trees. They were intimidating both in their girth and height.

Several of the trees were given names—"Colonel Armstrong," for example, is 308 feet tall and 15 feet in diameter. It was awesome to stand beside the Colonel and a few others. He is estimated to be about 1,400 years old. We thought about what the world was experiencing when the Colonel was a seedling. The Vikings hadn't invaded Europe and Ireland yet. It would be more than another hundred years before the marauders would wield their battle axes on the skulls of the Irish monks. The Colonel was already more than two hundred years old when Charlemagne arrived on the scene, rescuing the surviving Irish monks that illuminated the Dark Ages of the European continent, through preservation of historical documents, books, and their own writings.

We had our souvenir photos and an envelope of redwood seeds we bought at the little retail shop in the park grounds. The seeds were $1.50. We joked that it would be interesting to plant them at our golfing community home. What a sight that would be for golfers several hundred years from now—no shortcuts by hitting over the top of our tree to cut across the left-hand dogleg turn in the fairway.

For best results, the directions suggested refrigerating the seeds for thirty days. Soak overnight and allow plenty of room to grow. We kept the little packet in the fridge and every time we opened the door, it reminded us of our latest trip to California and that rustic little B&B. I have wonderful memories of the moments I spent with the sweetest and most delightful woman I ever met. She was a natural at it!

08/16/2008: My oldest stepson proposed to his girlfriend, Irene, in front of the castle at Disney's Magic Kingdom! Romantic, just like his father. Tom's son surprised Irene and went down on one knee. We had a grand party at the house. Tom and I went shopping for decorations and food. Bride and groom hats. Beautiful ring. Tom's sister and family came. More friends, neighbors, gifts, plenty of food and drink. I enjoyed getting ready for it. Very romantic.—I. C.

I couldn't ask for a more wonderful daughter-in-law. She is beautiful, too. The theme colors were black and white: balloons, crepe bands, and wedding bells strung throughout the downstairs. We had a big cake, but the happy couple didn't smash a piece in each other's face. That would have to wait for the wedding reception, in a little less than two years.

Tommy and Irene stayed at our home for a few more days before they had to get back to their normal work-a-day routines. Irene—my Irene—and I were very happy to host their party, and she was enthusiastic in all the preparations. She never complained. All she did was express how happy she was that my son was engaged to such a terrific young lady.

09/09/2008: Last clinic appointment until September 30. We continue leucovorin and 5-FU at home. The medical team is encouraging us to take the trip to Ireland. They want us to make sure we take snapshots of the sights. No one from our team has ever been there, and a couple of them are very interested.—I. C.

Erin Go Bragh—Cead Mille Failte!

Long Live Ireland—a Hundred Thousand Welcomes! Don't worry; I don't intend to turn this book into a travelogue, but I want to devote a few pages to a bit of our leisure time. Irene's ordeal became a lot more complicated and demanding as the months passed beyond this particular jaunt and our attempt to grasp some little pieces of life.

We again started planning for a trip in between infusions. We wanted to go to Ireland. By this time, we both felt capable of handling a trip overseas. Of course, we had to skip a chemo session one week so we could manage about ten days to two weeks away. There were a couple of days in travel time alone. We were glad that our medical team strongly supported the idea. The middle of September was a great time to fly to Ireland—fewer tourists. Irene looked forward to it, even though her chemo sessions left her just a little ragged around the edges.

Maria stayed in Bradenton while we toured. But before we left, Irene cooked some special meals for Maria and me. One of the family favorites was king crab legs with drawn butter. Irene cooked them perfectly every time. They were never tough. Maria sometimes ate at least a pound of them at a sitting. Irene and I could almost equal that amount, but Maria usually outlasted us. Irene's lobster tails were always delicious, too.

In preparation for our trip, we bought a couple travel guides and books. Rick Steves' paperback *Ireland 2008,* Avalon Travel Publishing, has a very concise history of Ireland from 7000 BC up to the publication date in 2008. I'm sure a more recent edition is in the bookstores now. It includes several detailed maps, an absolute necessity while touring Ireland, especially by car. In total, there are more than four hundred pages depicting just about every point of interest on the entire island, plus the islands that lay off the steep and craggy cliffs of the shoreline.

I mentioned the "famine" of 1932–33 in the Ukraine and the fact that it was contrived by the Soviet authorities. I also mentioned the similarities between the Ukrainian and Irish struggles for independence and their separate reactions to their cultural and historic plights. So in Irish history, from the Middle Ages forward, the English were the bad guys. To many fervent Irish nationalists, they still are to this day. The Potato Famine of 1845–49 is called by the nationalists, the "Great Hunger." Britain ruled the island at the time and was the wealthiest kingdom in the Western world, if not the entire world. England was accused of standing on the sidelines while more than a million Irish souls starved to death.

The famine caused a mass of emigrants to flee to the United States and elsewhere, into the arms of Lady Liberty. My grandmother came here in 1905 at the age of fourteen. I remember her telling us stories relating family "troubles" of her own great-grandparents' difficulty during the famine. She was a terrific storyteller. She had the gift of gab, as the Irish say, especially when she was in her cups.

The twenty-six counties that comprise the Republic of Ireland in the south have been free and independent of the crown since 1949. Not so for the six counties of Northern Ireland that remain part of the British system, although they operate as freely as, say, Canada. Rick Steves' summary is brief, almost up-to-date, and interesting.

The bastions of the occupying British military in the North were still evident along the border, with their machine guns and helmets, between the two parts of the Emerald Isle when I went there in 1976, on my first honeymoon. I drove up to the partition but turned around toward the south and friendlier rolling green hills.

In September 2008, Irene and I had more important interests in our lives than Irish history: touring and mingling with my ancestral relatives.

We landed at Shannon Airport and picked up our rental car. It took a few minutes to get used to the steering wheel being on the passenger's side of the front seats and a few more to re-familiarize myself driving on the wrong side of the road. I had done it before in 1976, and would do it again in 2010 with my son Chris.

Americans must be very careful when stepping off a curb into the street in Ireland. The traffic is coming from the opposite direction than here in the States. Irene had a very close call.

We booked most of our overnight lodging but decided to wing it on occasion. That is bad planning during the high season, but in mid- to late September, we had no trouble at all finding quaint little B&Bs.

We reserved the Bunratty Hotel the first couple of days and nights. The first day we drove into nearby Limerick. I snapped Irene's picture as she stood between two Irish police women patrolling the calm streets. King John's Castle was in the background.

The Bunratty Castle was a few hundred yards away from the hotel. It features a medieval feast, complete with traditional Irish music, including harp and fiddle. Ireland boasts three castles that present the fare local kings and court followers enjoyed during those olden days. When in Ireland, participating in that atmosphere should be mandatory. When I review the photos and videos from the Bunratty Castle feast, I am so happy to see Irene laughing and smiling with wide-eyed delight, as she sang along with well-known Irish songs. The entertainers stir the feasting revelers to sing as loudly as they can. Irene's soul was revealing itself. Mine too!

We drove the narrow roads through the "terrible beauty" of the Burren toward the coast. The Burren is a barren, rocky no-man's-land, to which farmers from the rest of Ireland were exiled by the English royalty of the time. Their family farms were confiscated and given to crown loyalists. Also on the west coast, rising almost seven hundred feet out of the depths of the Atlantic Ocean, we stood on the brink of the Cliffs of Moher and held our breath.

Then we motored onward and upward to Galway Bay and its suburb Claddagh, which claims to be the birthplace of the famous engagement/wedding rings that Irene and I both wear. Galway is a university town with lots of street entertainment. Harp tones bounce from every building. Student performers continually strum that national symbol, a favorite musical instrument for many Irishmen. We heard its soothing vibrations and the floating sounds of tin whistles around every corner we turned in the outdoor market area. We dined in local pubs and when in Ireland, I drank Guinness beer with our hearty meals.

In Cong and nearby, we visited a re-creation of the thatched roof home John Wayne had in his terrific role in *Quiet Man*, the movie. And we had to have tea and scones on the grounds of Ashford Castle where the rich and famous lodge while visiting Ireland. Inside Ashford Castle, the mahogany walls, intricately designed tapestries, and crystal chandeliers combine to just exude elegance. We had a very nice taste of it and then continued on our way.

Further north, we stayed over in Westport, County Mayo, which we used as a headquarters to venture an hour or two both eastward and westward. Just outside of town is St. Patrick's Croagh, his mountain. Eastward brought us to the Shrine of Knock, where we attended mass celebrated in the ancient Gaelic language.

We collected holy water at Knock to bring home. Then we drove to Achill Island off the coast of County Mayo, my ancestral county. Just over the causeway is a little cemetery with possibly two hundred headstones. Under at least 20 percent of those grave markers lay the remains of a Cooney, several named Thomas. I took photos of names and dates. I had a private thought as I looked at all those grave markers.

What were their final thoughts? Did Danny Boy kneel reverently beside one of these weathered tombstones? Which one? I wonder.

Continuing our scenic drive along the scary coastline roads to the end of Achill Island, we found a beach, probably straight across the ocean from Boston. The water was beautiful but cold. We dipped our toes and climbed back up the steep incline to the road. Even my videos of that winding narrow drive are still frightening but gorgeous.

Then we drove straight southeastward to Tara, the Hill of Kings and of Scarlet O'Hara fame. It's near the scene of the historic Battle of Boyne in 1690, when Protestants defeated the Catholics. For the next three hundred years, the Catholics were a subjugated minority under British rule. Even their music was outlawed.

Close by Tara and the Boyne River are ancient prehistoric ruins. Ireland has been inhabited at least as far back as 7000 BC and has extensive archeological evidence of that very early culture.

We bypassed Dublin, founded by the Vikings, and went straight southward. In 1976, my former wife and I toured "Ireland's fair city, where the girls are so pretty." I thought that the hustle and bustle would be too tiring for us to do a visit any justice. Time restraints were beginning to rule too. Dublin and its environs is an area a couple should spend at least a week touring. We still had a place or two to visit, and there would be a lot of miles to transverse across the south of the island. The southern coast, with all its long-standing fishing villages, was a wonderful little route for lunchtime and dinnertime stops along the way to Cork and Blarney Castle.

Kissing the Blarney Stone endows you with the gift of gab, according to legend. The gift includes a disarming and smiling eloquence. Irish diplomacy, a resultant trait for kissing the stone, is "the ability to tell someone to go to hell so that he is looking forward to the trip." Some people wouldn't dare kiss the Blarney Stone—hyper-scared of germs. Others go to Ireland and don't care if they do anything else as long as they kiss the stone. Irene and I belonged to the "must do" group—we kissed it! Irene kissed it carefully. She risked it. It was too important. We also had tea and scones on the grounds of the castle.

Over in Killarney, if you describe the four peninsulas as fingers that jut westward out into the Atlantic Ocean in southwest Ireland, we were situated at the knuckles. We needed much more time to drive around all four fingers. We didn't do them all. We chose the Ring of Kerry. For most of the day, we were treated with views of magnificent rough seas and craggy cliffs all along the narrow roads. At the beginning and the end of our tour was Killarney, with all its horse-drawn carriages. We stayed in another B&B with a panoramic view of the area. The owner made the best Irish breakfast we ate on the whole trip. Breakfast is included at most B&Bs. We couldn't stomach the blood pudding, though. I just had to deliver a pun again.

On the ride back to Limerick, we took a ferry ride. That was fun. People use it every day to go back and forth to work. It sails at least every hour. During peak times, when two boats were running, the passengers could catch a ride every half hour.

We returned to Limerick to a hotel we'd booked before we left home. We wanted to be near the airport because our flight left early in the morning. The motif was aeronautical, with paintings and photographs of famous pilots, including Amelia Earhart and Howard Hughes. The pictures were hung all over the walls in the lobby and suites. A short drive took us to Adare, a village of thatched homes, tearooms, and fiddlers on the street. We had a couple Irish beers in one of the pubs and toasted each other.

"*Slainte*, Tom."

"'Tis the Irish in ye risin' to the soorface is it, colleen?"

"Aye, 'deed 'tis, sire! Will ye be 'avin' a scone wit yer tea, 'andsome?"

"I will, me beauty!"

Once home, we arranged our next chemo appointment. The fun and freedom was over for now. Reality hit us again. The next part of our journey would demand all the hope and strength Irene could muster.

The Struggle Continues

We returned from Ireland on September 26, 2008, in time to make our next appointment to continue chemo. We saw the oncologist four days later on September 30.

09/30/2008: Filled in the team on our trip. Resumed my regular chemo infusions, FOLFIRI plus Avastin. Will start tomorrow.–I. C.

As of October 1, Irene continued infusions through her port with 5-FU, leucovorin, and irinotecan (FOLFIRI), plus Avastin. She had received FOLFIRI for the last four months, with a one-week delay, when we flew to California and then another week delay for the Ireland trip. Irene and I would occasionally go out to dinner when she felt up to it. We held hands across the table. Life seemed normal for a little while.

According to the scans, Irene's cancer was "indolent"; that is, not getting worse. I always thought indolent meant "lazy." The nuns used it a lot when I was a kid, as in, "You, Master Cooney, are an indolent little street urchin"—I think that was in second grade. In fact, indolent also is a medical term.

11/12/2008: Normal visit. Continue neulasta injection twenty-four hours after the 5-FU is disconnected at home to help keep white blood cell count normal. Can't do chemo if white cell count is too low. End table and dresser is full of meds. Dr. Tom gives me the shot along with the blood thinner.—I. C.

Irene handled the pain and discomfort well. The persistent fatigue, abdominal discomfort, migraines, and tingling in her fingers, however, were still a nuisance. Life was as good as it could be, under the circumstances, for a couple weeks, until …

12/07/2008: Tom rushed me to local hospital ER. I was admitted immediately from ER. They could tell I was really in agony. I was having severe pain in my abdomen and blood in my stool and high fever. After many tests, doctors say it may be a virus that is going around. Many people having same symptoms. Pain meds administered through IV along with antibiotics.—I. C.

Cancer patients are more prone to infection, due to the side effects caused by some chemo protocols—reduced white blood cell count (neutropenia), for example. We were careful to avoid exposure to infection.

12/11/2008: The local doctors couldn't find any cause. Kept for observation and diagnostic tests. Unknown diagnosis. Symptoms subsided. Discharged after four days.—I. C.

In upcoming years, I rushed Irene to our preferred local hospital emergency room four times for various conditions. Those emergency visits resulted in two admissions, including the one Irene just noted at that particular hospital and two follow-up admissions at Moffitt.

Those biweekly sessions took us through the Thanksgiving holidays into December. We went to Bradenton for Thanksgiving and again tried to make it a two-fer by stopping at my sister's on the way home. Also, during the holidays, our families watched all our videos from Ireland.

We had an appointment in the GI clinic on December 22. Irene had lost about five pounds since the last visit. In consideration of the recent hospital stay a couple weeks earlier, plus the "cumulative effects of ongoing toxicity" for several months with just a few one week infusion delays, the team decided to give her a treatment holiday. Her blood work was acceptable to permit the break too.

Irene and I welcomed the vacation, especially over the holidays. The next appointment for restaging scans and blood work was in February 2009. Restless, we visited Bradenton and my sister's family during the nervous interim.

In the meantime, we kept an appointment with our local doctor. Irene was experiencing a little bit of discomfort in her lower back and hips.

01/03/09: Tom took me to our family doctor. Bone density scan of hip and spine ordered by family doctor. Mild osteoporosis left hip. Treated with meds: Fusomax 70 mg.—I. C.

Another Disappointment

02/07/2009: Enjoyed the holidays. Started chemo again. (FOLFIRI) with Avastin (bevacizumab)—no oxaliplatin, thank God.—I. C.

After that welcome break from infusions, Irene started the sessions again, primarily for ongoing maintenance. But she could hardly get out of bed all week after that session. It was unexpected because the cocktail didn't contain her nemesis drug, oxaliplatin. She was vomiting all the time. She was extremely fatigued and had severe diarrhea.

02/17/2009: I've been in bed since I had chemo on the seventh. Really feeling miserable. Scans next week.—I. C.

02/25/2009: The latest scans showed new lesion in my liver and activity near my right lower lung—I had surgery there. I hope it didn't come back there. I was asked by a member of the team if I wanted to stop chemo—you know, the "quality" thing. I do not want to stop. I can handle it. I don't like the alternative. Went upstairs to infusion room in wheelchair. I got one of the private beds in one of the "penthouses." Continued chemo again with reduced doses. They gave me atropine and antihistamine before the cocktail. Tom kissed me nighty-night, and I slept through six hours of infusion. I needed the sleep. Tom wandered the halls. We'll go back to GI clinic for assessment in a couple weeks.—I. C.

A new lesion was detected in her liver. Chemo restarted so her nausea increased and the fatigue, as usual, got worse. Diarrhea was very bothersome, as you can imagine. The usual side effects intensified.

03/11/2009: Received my FOLFIRI plus Avastin infusion. Still a reduced dose from the first one I got this year in early February. Nausea, vomiting continues. Team told me they will present my case to the Tumor Board regarding if I'm a candidate for surgery again. We had discussed it before. This is a follow-up.—I. C.

03/27/2009: Continuing same regimen in reduced doses. Tom continuing neulasta shots at home for building white cells.—I. C.

04/08/2009: Doctor increased my Dilaudid Rx at my request. Pain in my stomach is really bad. Tom only one who really knows.—I. C.

05/13/2009: Hair falling out again. Staying on same cocktail. After infusion they hook up the 5-FU booster. At home, disconnect forty-six hours after. Home health nurse flushes and twenty-four hours later, Tom gives me the neulasta injection. We are praying. It's been almost six years.—I. C.

Huge Intersession

06/10/2009: Prayer counts! New scan is "excellent." Scan is great. Whoopee! Still have severe foot and hand pain, hair loss, constipation for a switch from the usual diarrhea. Team approved a two-month treatment break. Whoopee! Thank you, Lord, and St. Theresa!—I. C.

Another two months' treatment break! God heard! Irene could use a break, as long as it didn't impede recovery too much. We always fully understood our situation. Quality of life was really up to us. Quantity of life was the team's goal.

Irene was really ready for a break. And there is something romantic and exotic about taking a train trip. We agreed on "riding the rails" to Savannah.

"Whoopee! We're gonna take a train ride to Savannah. It'll be romantic."

"I'll get the tickets right away, honey. Maybe we'll meet famous people in the club car … or dining car … or sleeper car! Who do you remember most from all those scenes we've seen from the movies about the Orient Express and the Trans-Siberian Railroad, honey?"

"Peter Lorre … I think! But then there was Charlie Chan, too. Wasn't there?"

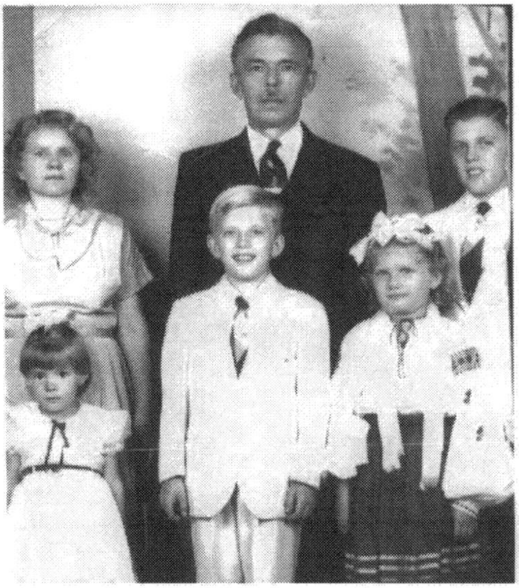

Irene, as the youngest of her four siblings (lower left). Maria, Irene's mom, is right behind Irene on the left in the back row.

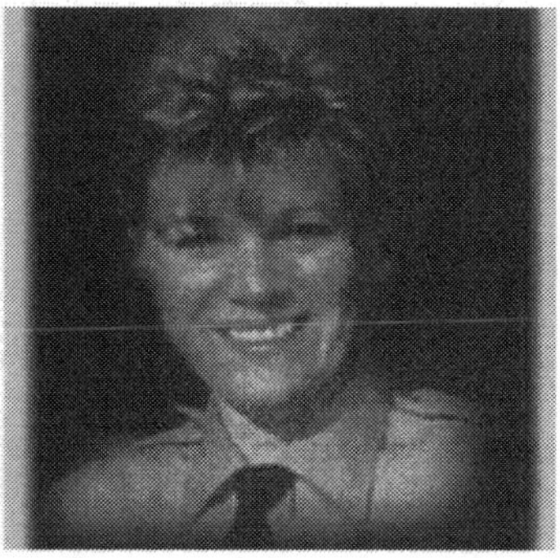

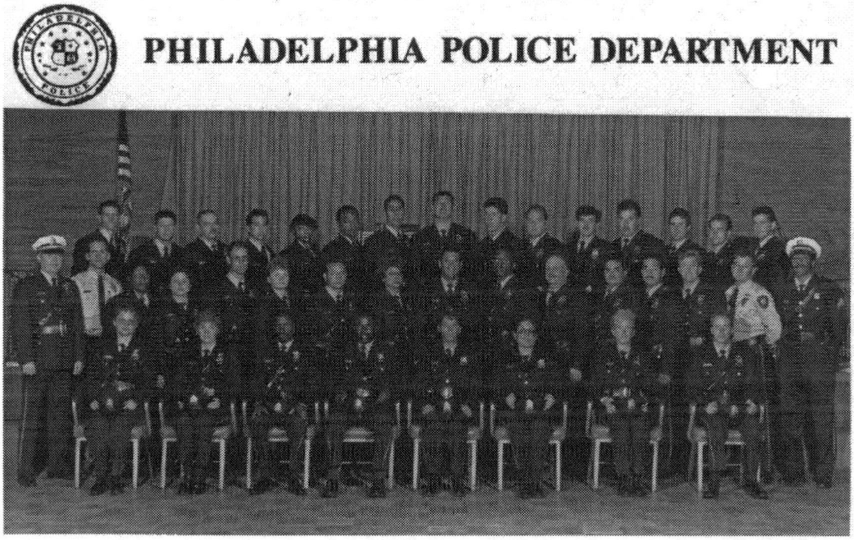

Irene is second from the left in first row. When Irene graduated from her Police Academy class, it was the start of a new life she had only dreamed about in the past. She was about 37 years old when she graduated in 1990.

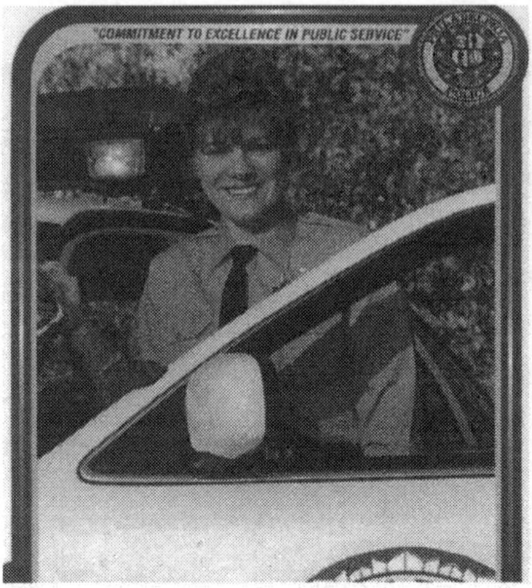

Irene on patrol, protecting the citizens of Philadelphia (1990)

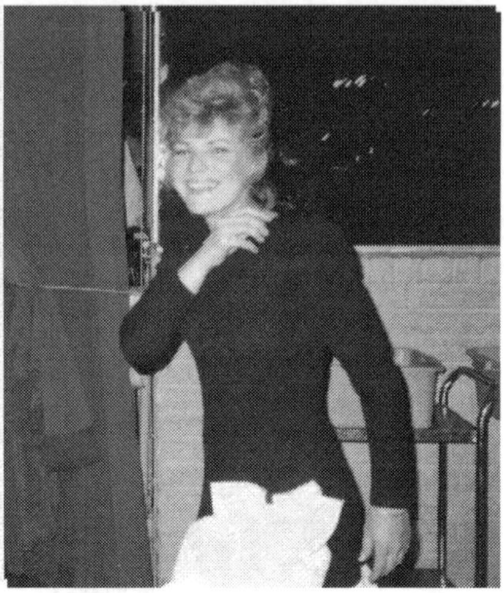

Look at that smile! Look at that figure, too!

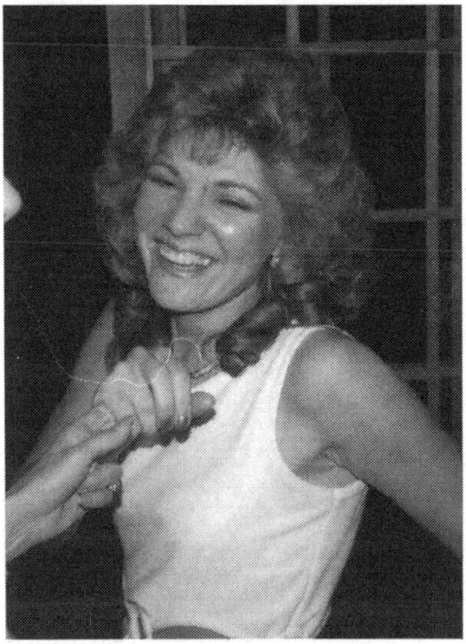

Irene during happier days (pre-diagnosis) with all her great hair.

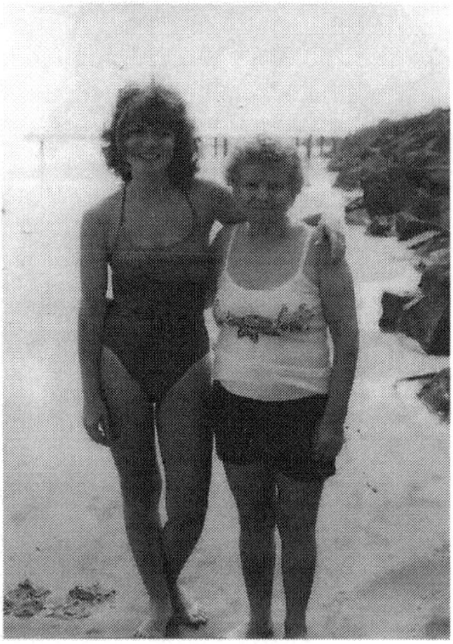

Irene and her mom, Maria, in the late '80s.

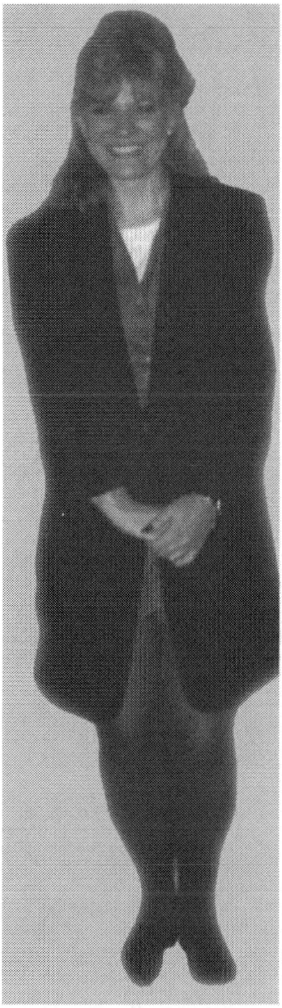

This is my favorite pose of Irene. It best portrays her personality. It's from a group photo of when Irene was assigned to the DA's office and had the alias of "Kathy Falcone" (ca. 2000).

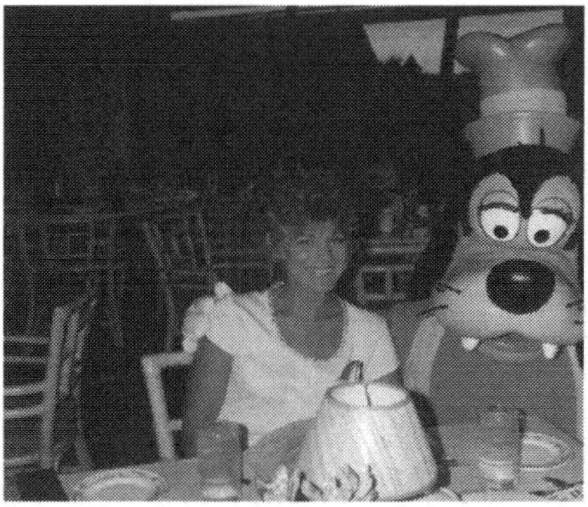

Irene with Goofy, above; with the Philly Phanatic, below.

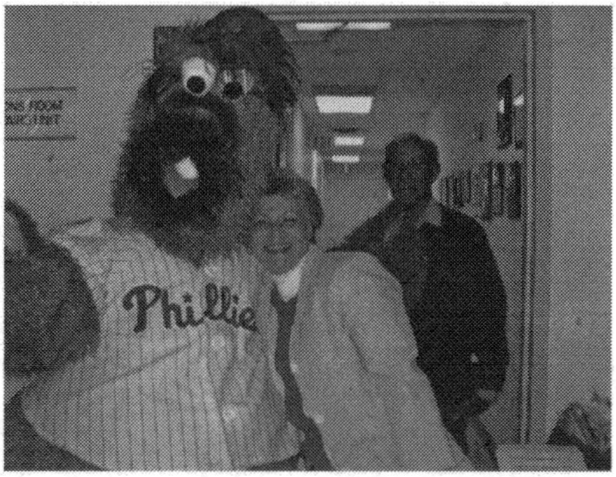

Below: Irene mimicking me while we were on one of our trips to Las Vegas. Her hair thinned a little bit by this time.

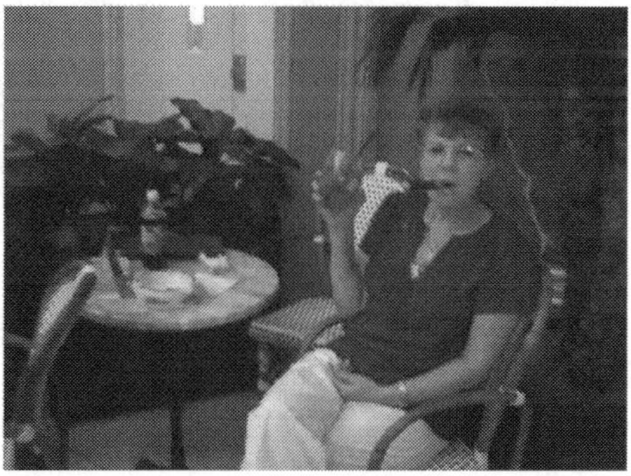

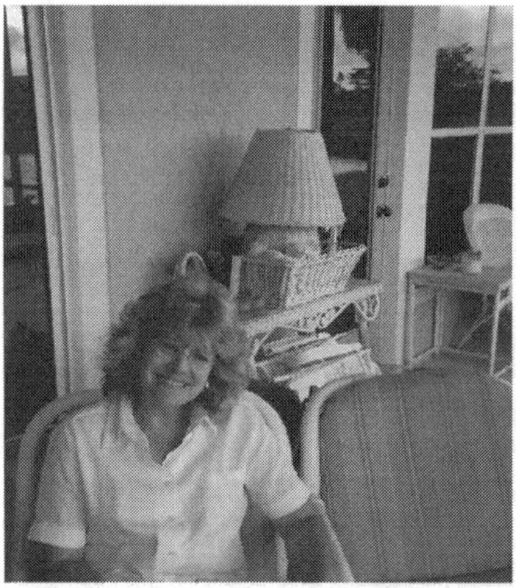

Enjoying the lanai on one of her first visits to the Florida home (2002). This is pre-cancer diagnosis.

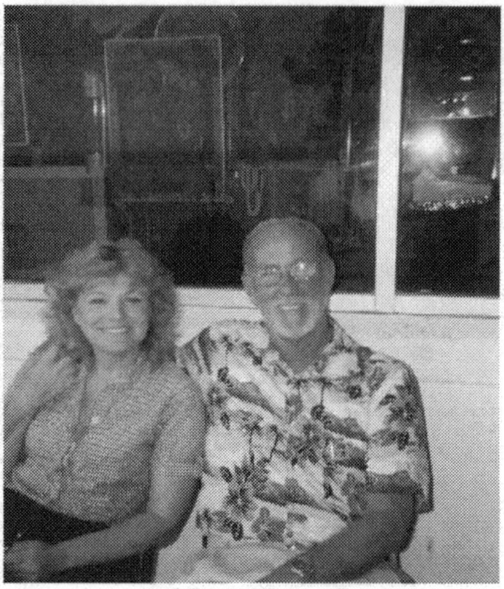

At a beachside café on Anna Maria Island near Bradenton on one of my first trips to Bradenton (2002).

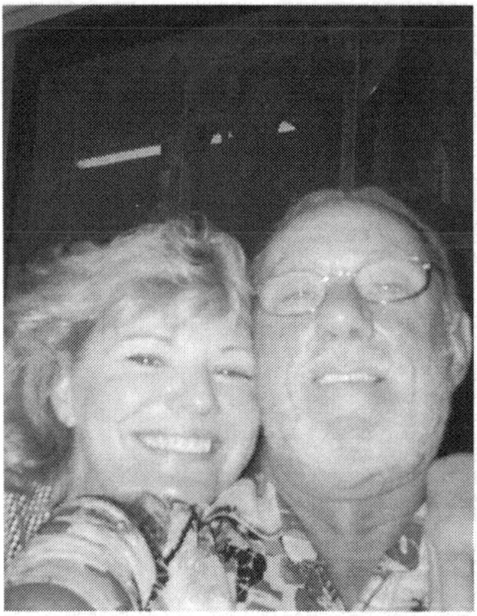

This is at the same beachside café as photo at upper right. I wanted to prove I could snap a self-photo.

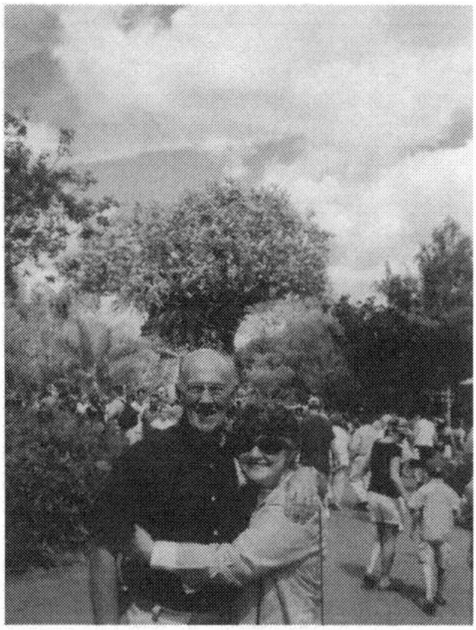

Here we are, ironically, at "The Tree of Life" in Disney World's Animal Kingdom.

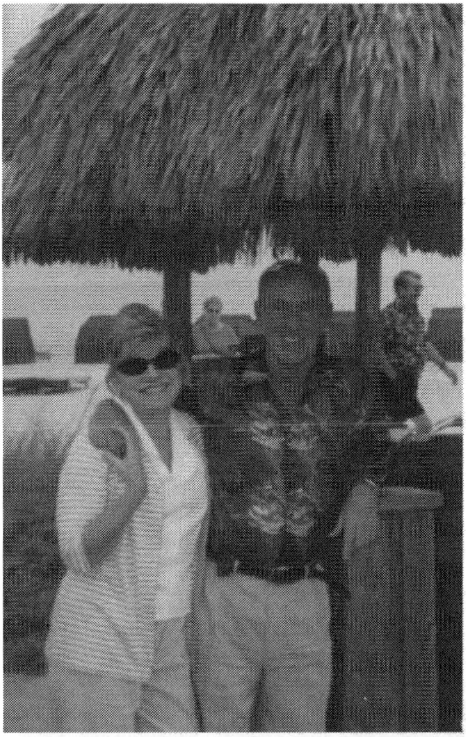

I couldn't resist showing you why Irene and I preferred Florida over Philly. In one photo we are on the beach during the winter of 2004-2005. A short time later, we are in Philly under different climatic conditions. That's Irene all bundled up.in the photo below. I'm under the deck looking out toward the rear driveway that we had to clear in order to get to the street.

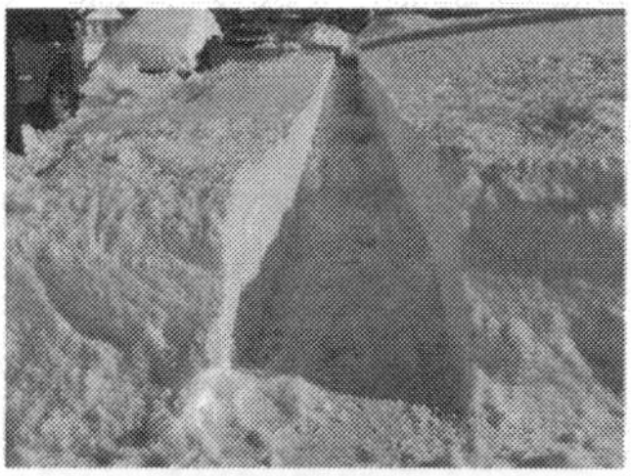

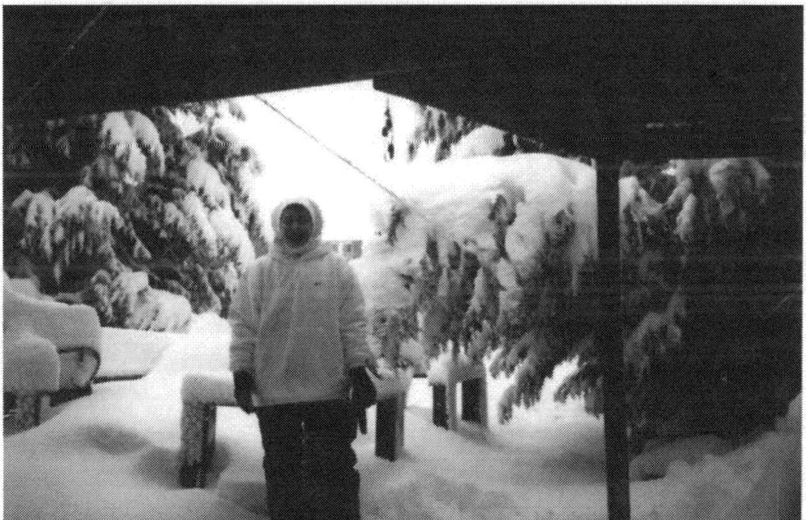

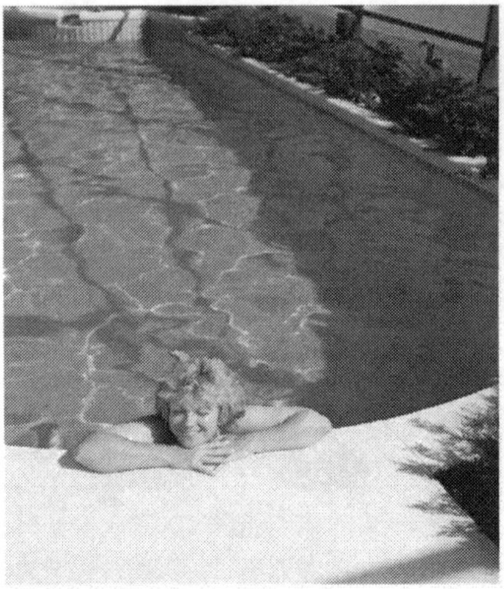

Skinny-dipping. There's nobody behind us or on either side.

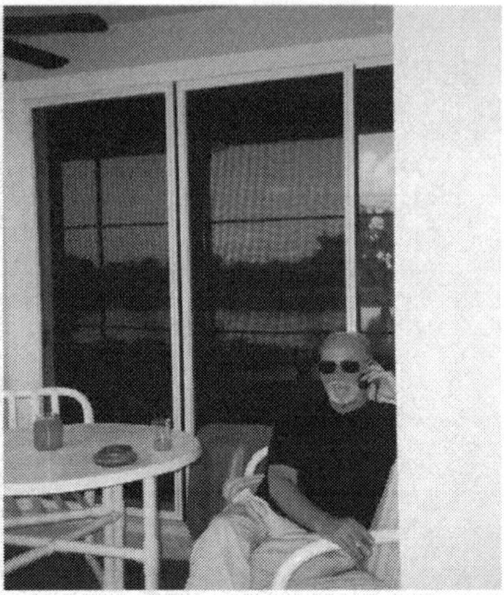

Me, watching Irene skinny-dip. I had a drink, a cigar, a cell, and sunglasses. What else is there?

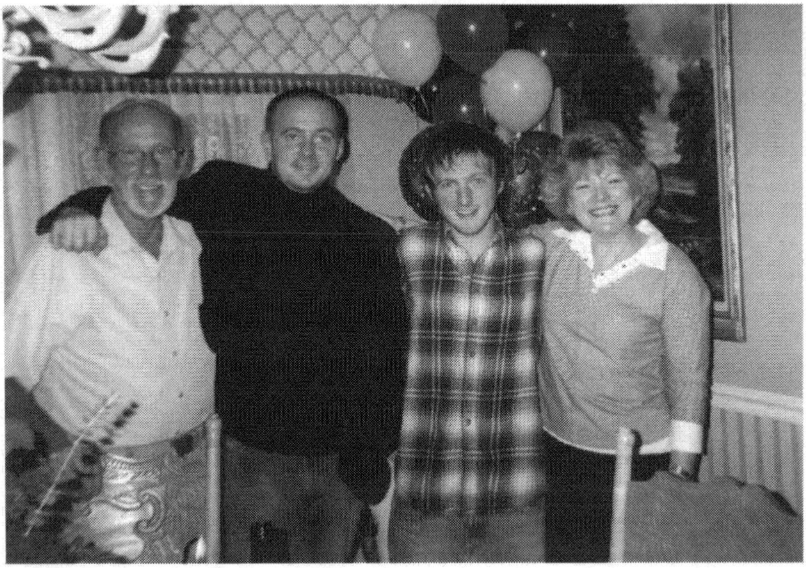

Me, my elder son, my younger son, and Irene, after having goose, Charles Dickens-style, at the Fox Chase home in Philadelphia. This photo was taken shortly after Irene's diagnosis in 2003. You can see that my belly is full.

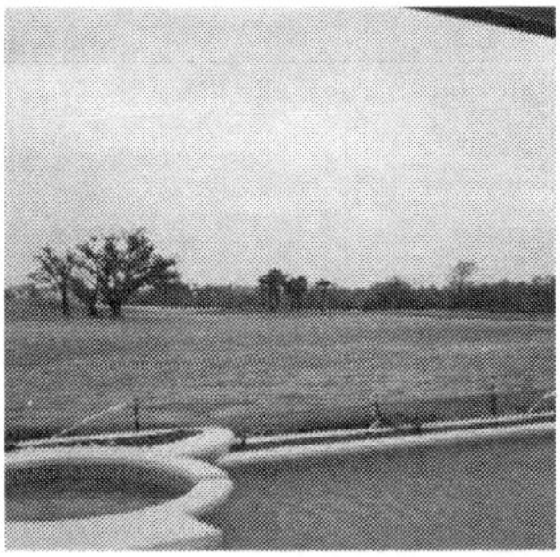

Hurricane '04. The rear-view without the pool screen and the pond over-flowing.

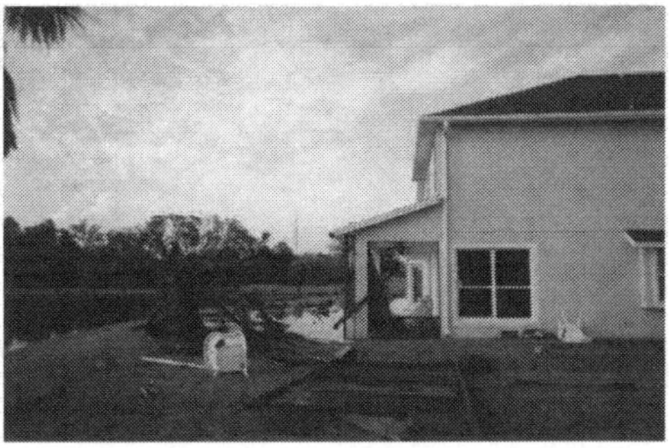

The pool screen was ripped out of the concrete base and strewn across the lawn. Irene battled this storm with me.

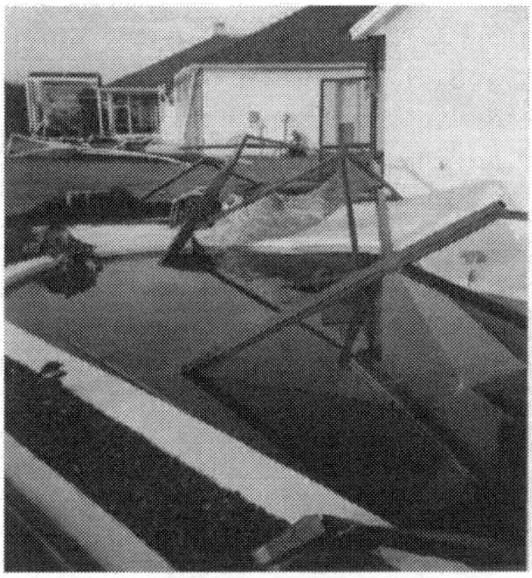

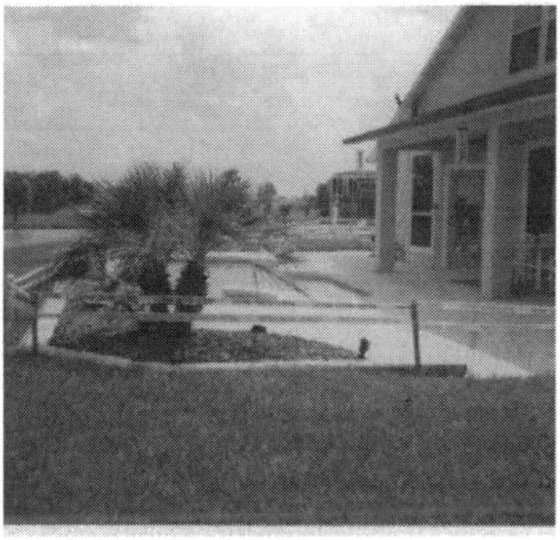

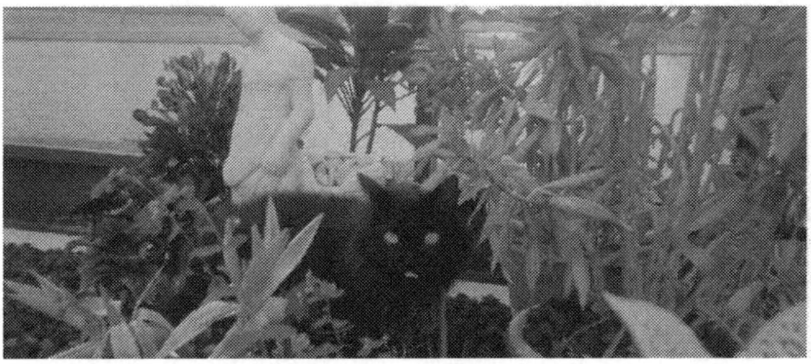

Dusty. He loved to stalk the big birds from inside the safety of the new pool screen.

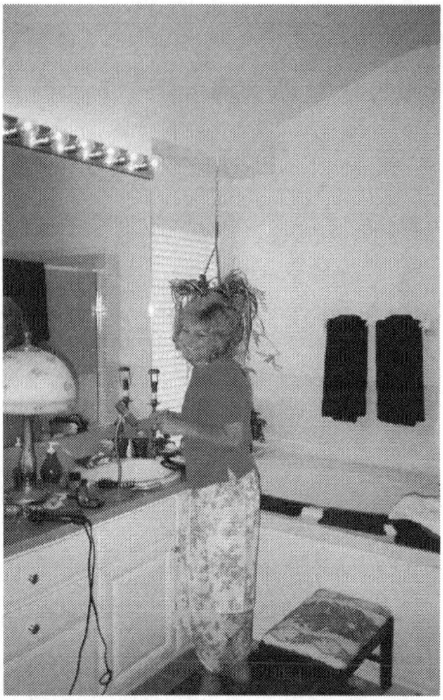

Irene getting ready for a trip to Savannah. We took the train to experience something different.

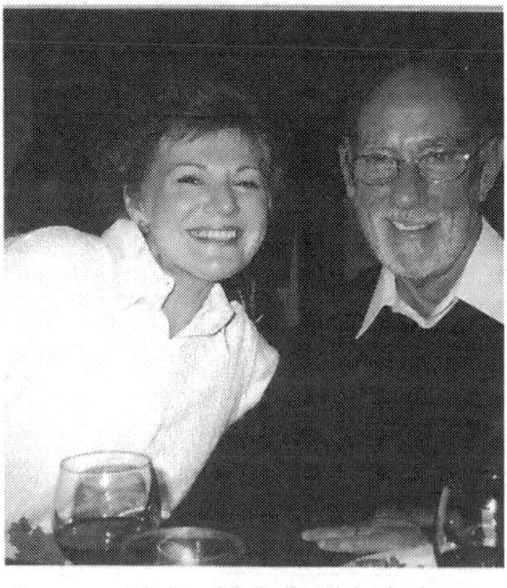

Irene with "rabbit fur" hairdo.

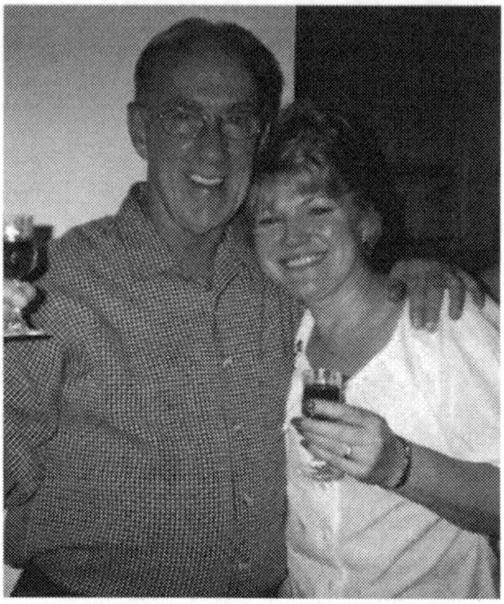

A happy couple enjoying some California wine in Savannah, GA. My networking niece arranged the room.

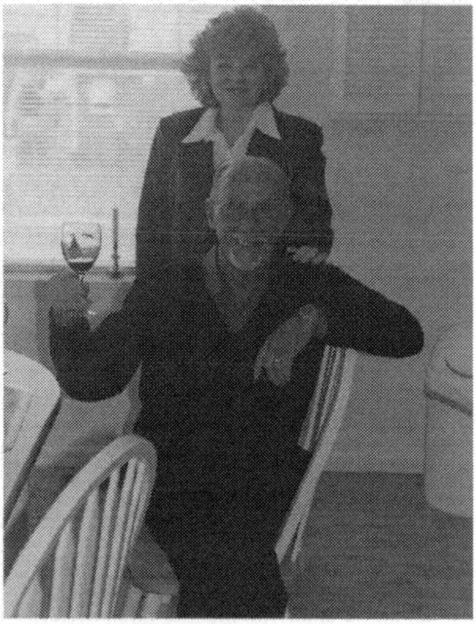

At my brother and sister-in-law's in Wildwood, NJ , circa 2008. Her hair had grown back again as it usually does.

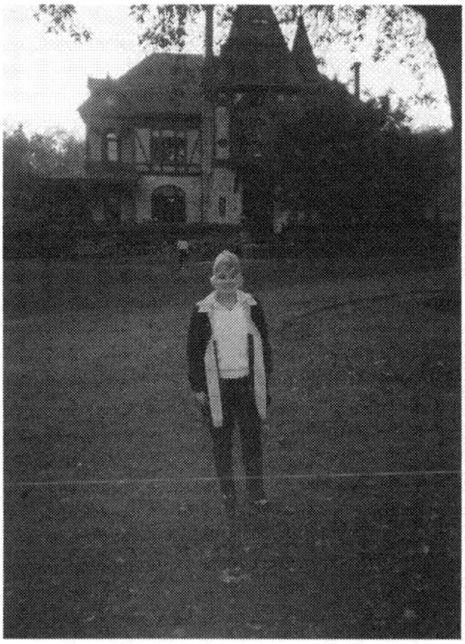

Francis Ford Coppola's winery in Napa Valley, California.

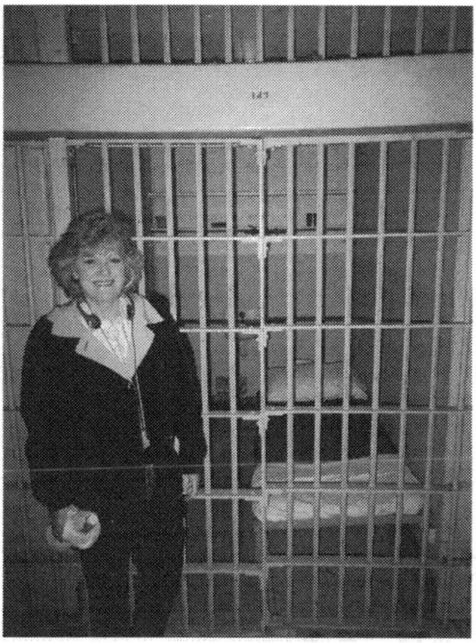

Al Capone's cell at Alcatraz. We took a quick trip to the "Rock."

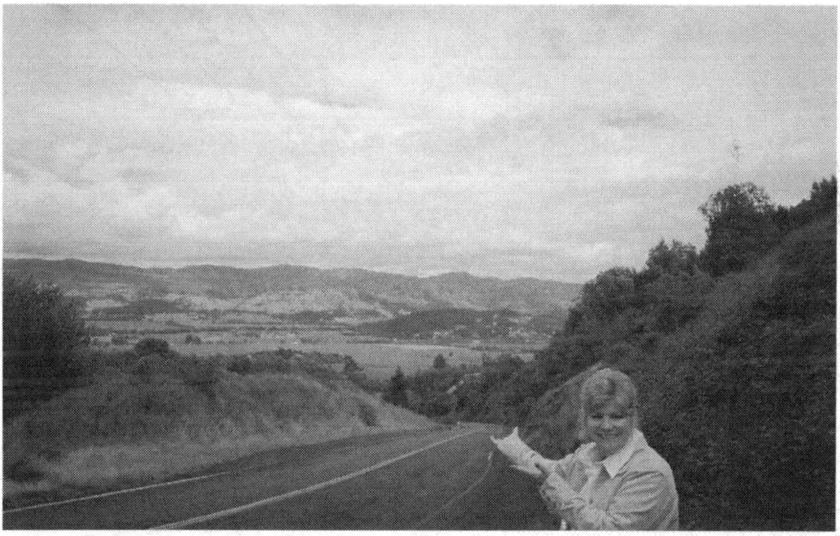

Irene showing everyone how to get from Sonoma Valley to Napa Valley through a shortcut. We wanted a last visit to Beringer's winery, our favorite in Napa Valley.

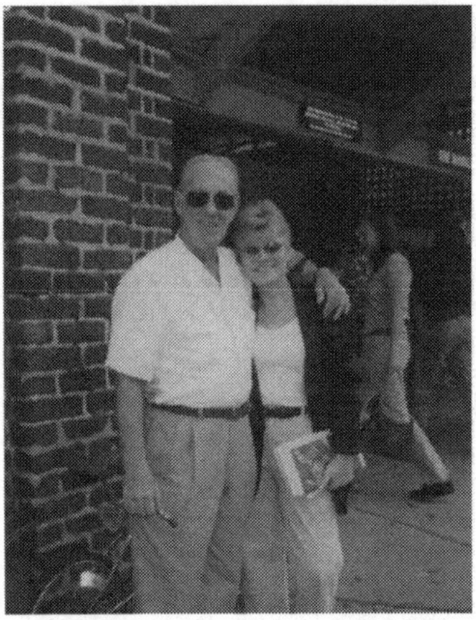

We often stopped in Charleston, SC, on our way to and from Florida.

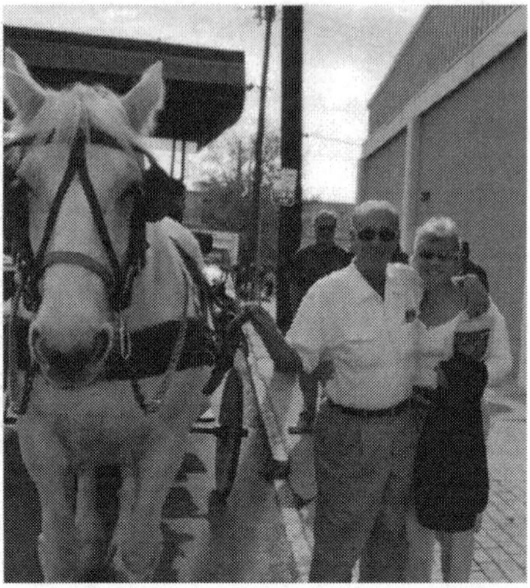

Irene enjoyed her first horse and carriage tour while in Charleston, SC.

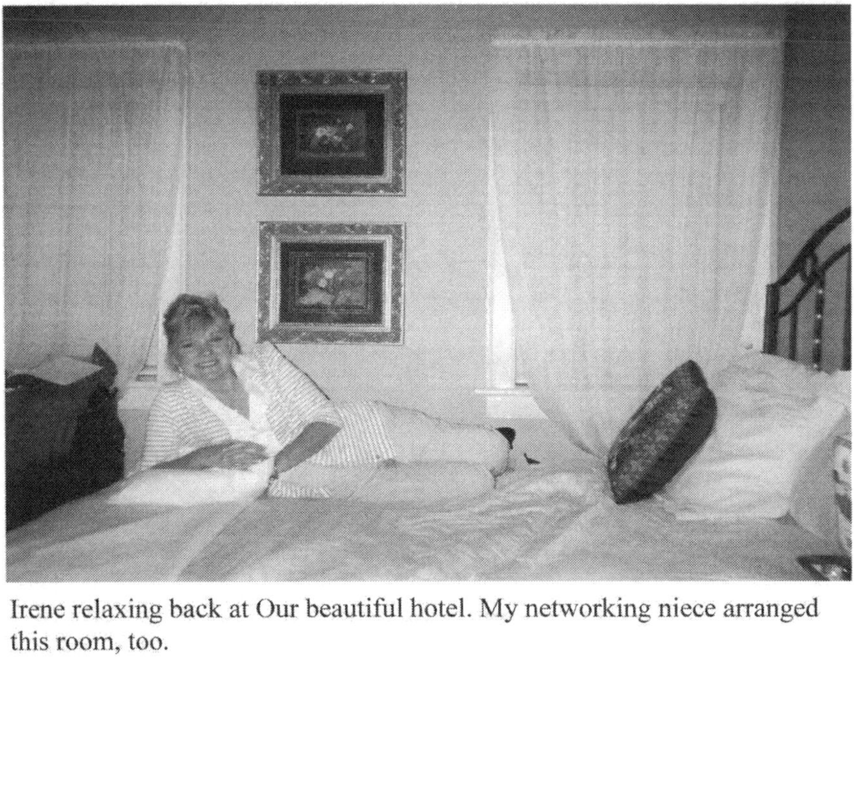

Irene relaxing back at Our beautiful hotel. My networking niece arranged this room, too.

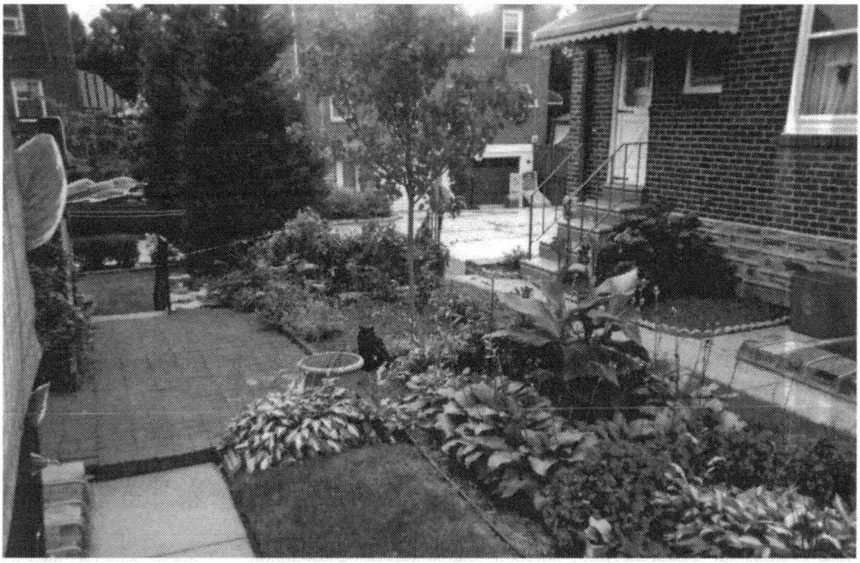

Dusty in the middle of Irene's breezeway garden in Fox Chase section of Philly. This house was very convenient to Fox Chase Cancer Center, only 10 minutes away. Dusty is sitting near where his two pals are buried. Does he sense their "presence"? What do you think?

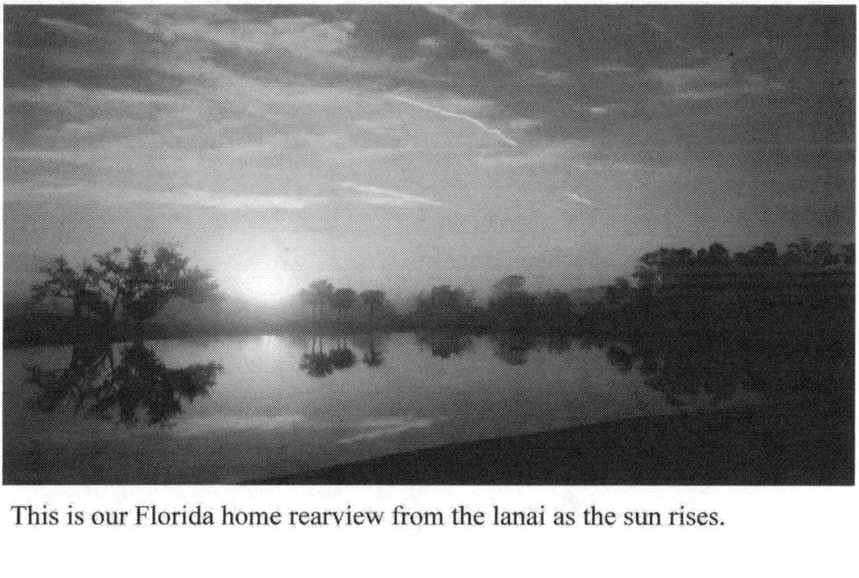

This is our Florida home rearview from the lanai as the sun rises.

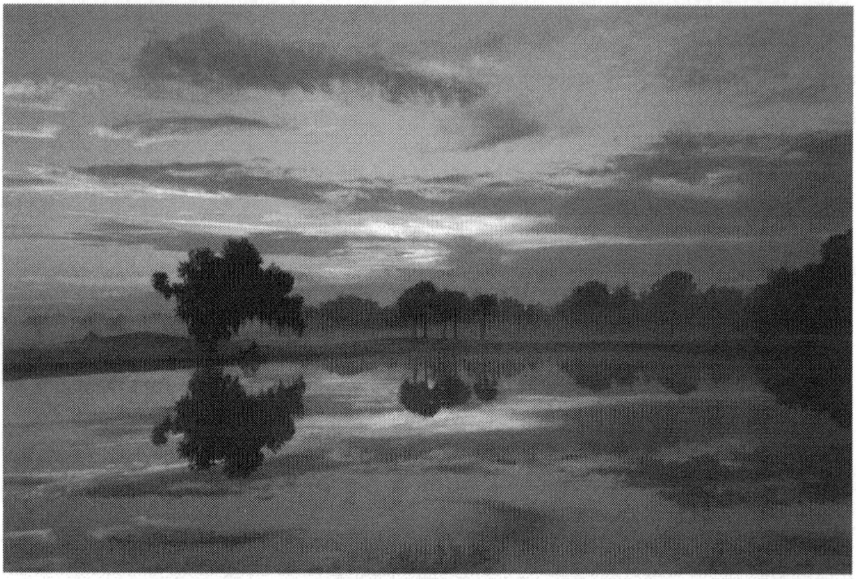

Irene loved to have her "cawfee" on the lanai and watch the sun come up. Every morning presented a different, but beautiful, scene. I probably have at least 50 photos from the same perspective yet all of them are unique. Irene and I regularly watched the sun rise.

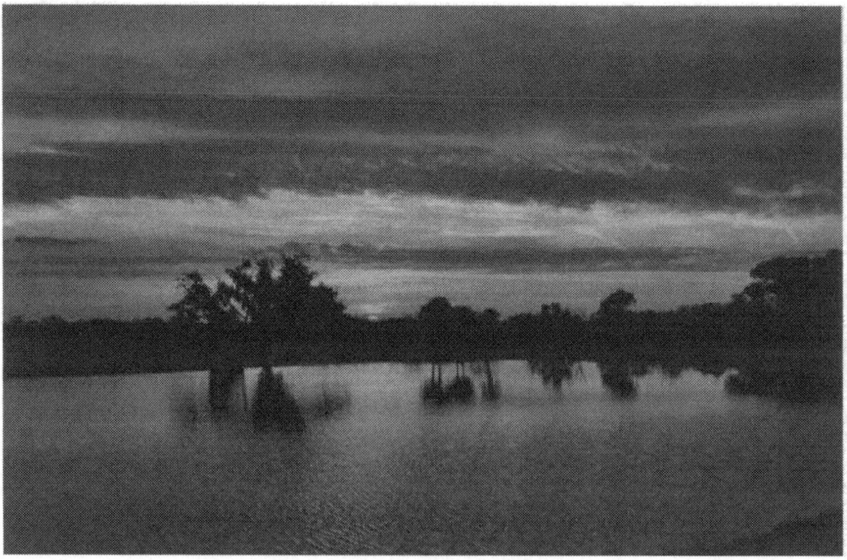

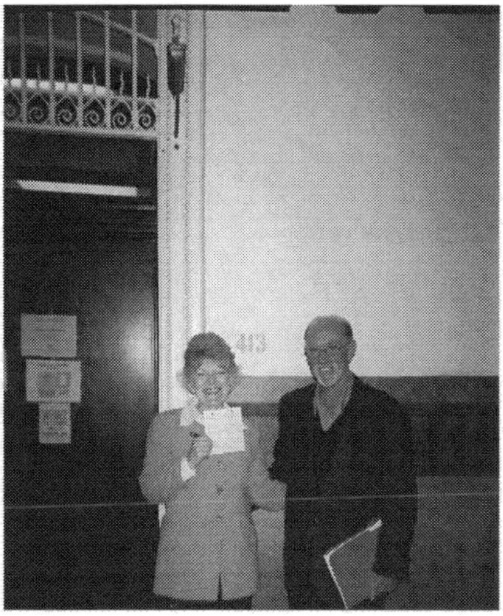

Picking up our marriage license at city hall in Philadelphia.

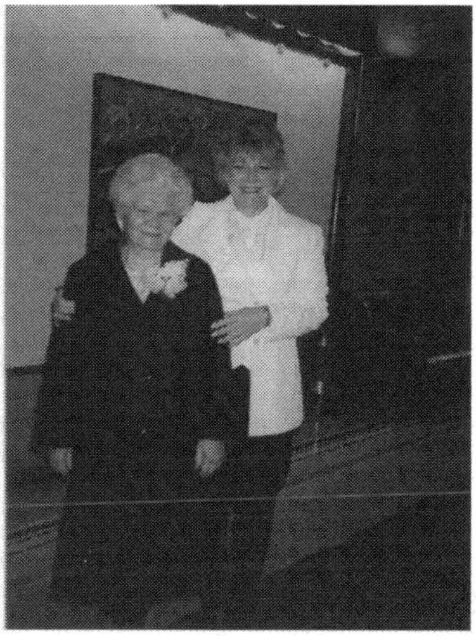

Irene and Maria on our wedding day.

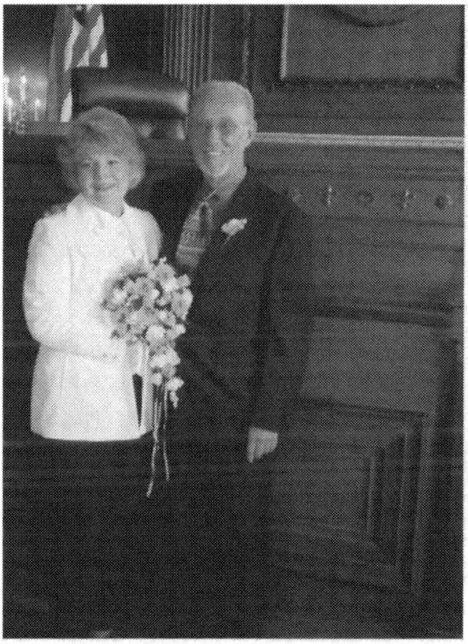

Newly weds: Mr. & Mrs. Cooney. 'Til death do us part. We had 7 more years.

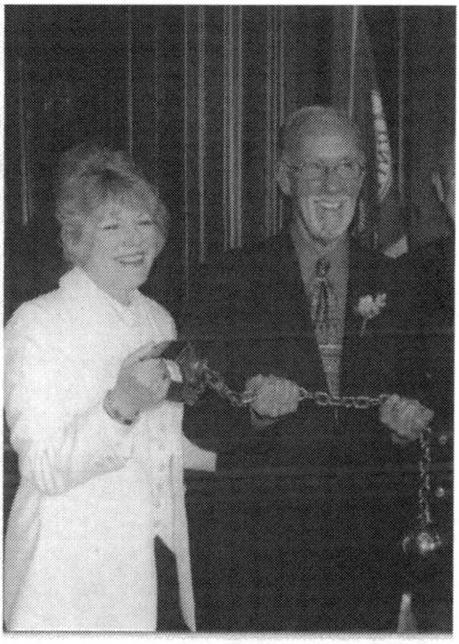

Irene and I with the ball and chain. I loved every minute of being shackled to Irene.

Wedding party. My brother and his wife on the left; Irene and me in the center; and, my two sons on the right.

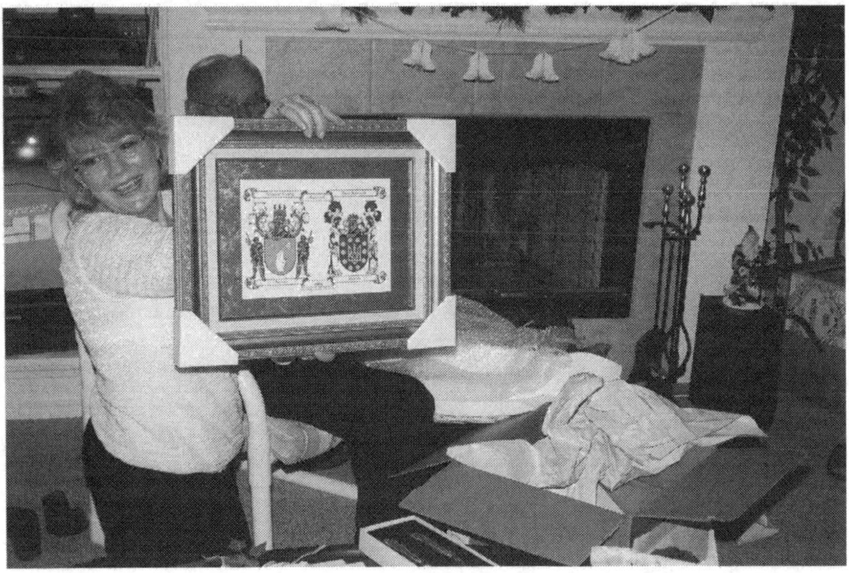

We had a reception at our home in Florida. The gift we show above is a beautifully framed "Cooney" Coat of Arms joined with the "Ukrainian" Coat of Arms. The couple who gave it to us are now both deceased.

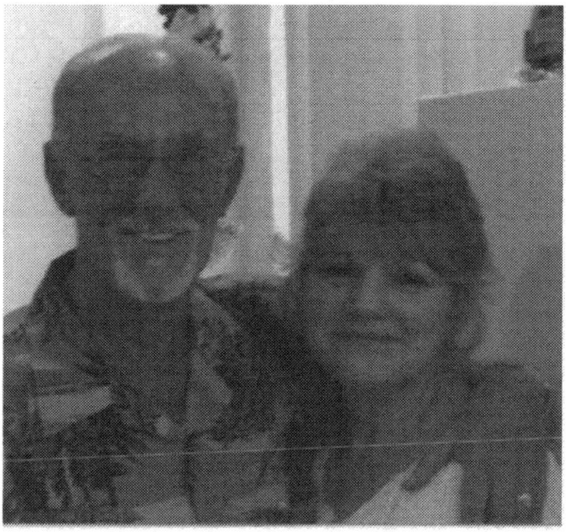

At our wedding reception when we returned to Florida. Don't we look happy? You can notice my Claddagh ring at the lower right.

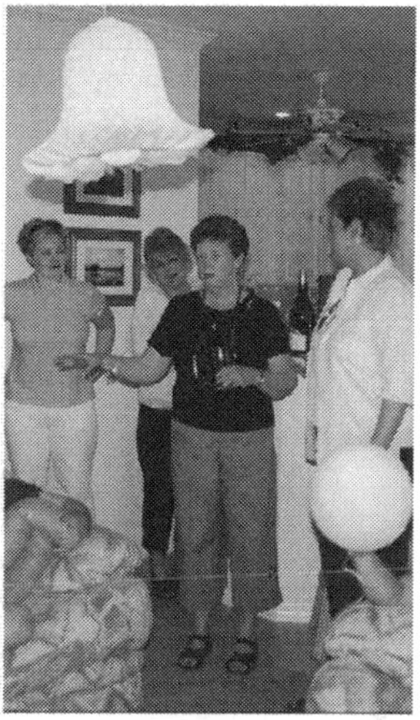

My sister and my nieces holding court with Irene looking on.

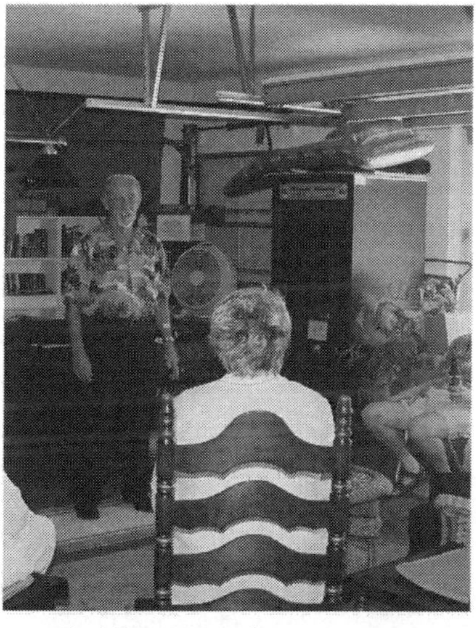

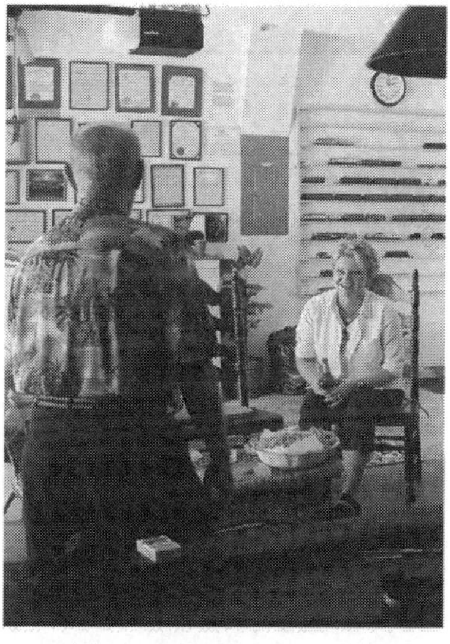

Me holding court in the garage during our wedding reception. I evidently got a laugh out of my networking niece.

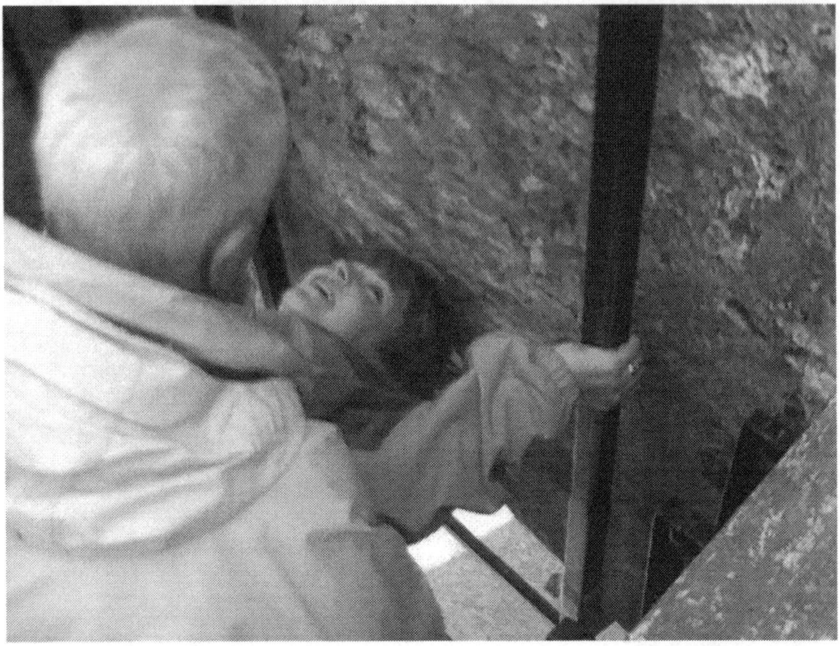

Kissing the Blarney Stone was a "Must Do" in Ireland for Irene. This was tough for Irene but she did it anyway.

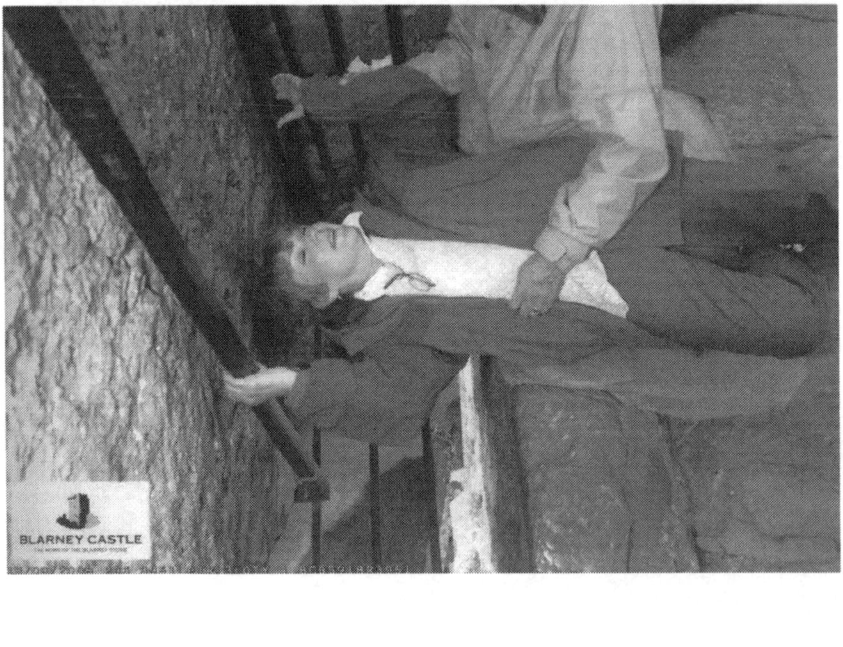

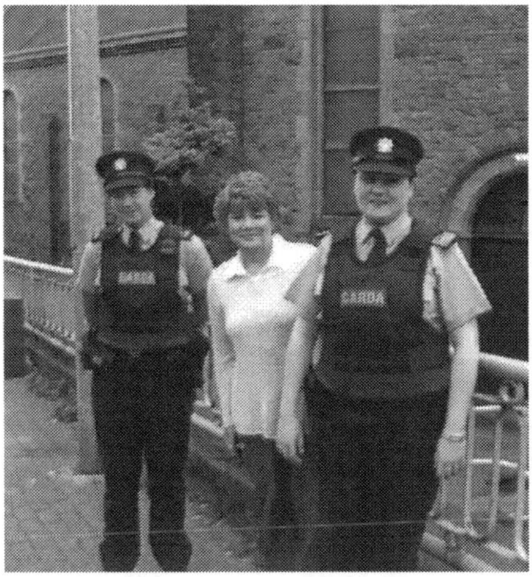

Trading war stories with a couple Irish policewomen.

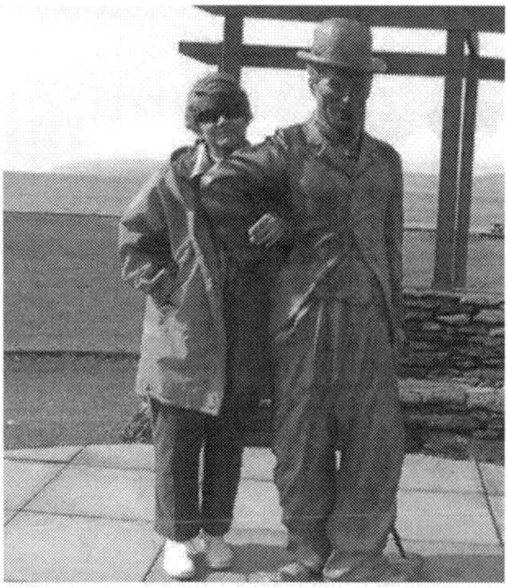

Irene & Charlie Chaplin during our tour of the Ring of Kerry.

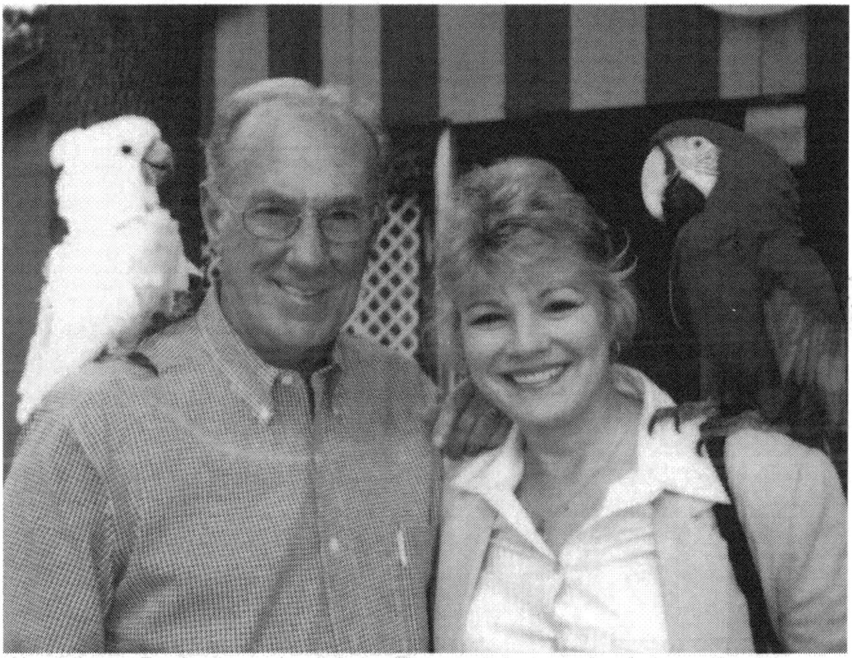

Back home in the Sunshine State after our trip to Ireland. Irene liked to visit the many flea markets in our area. So did I.

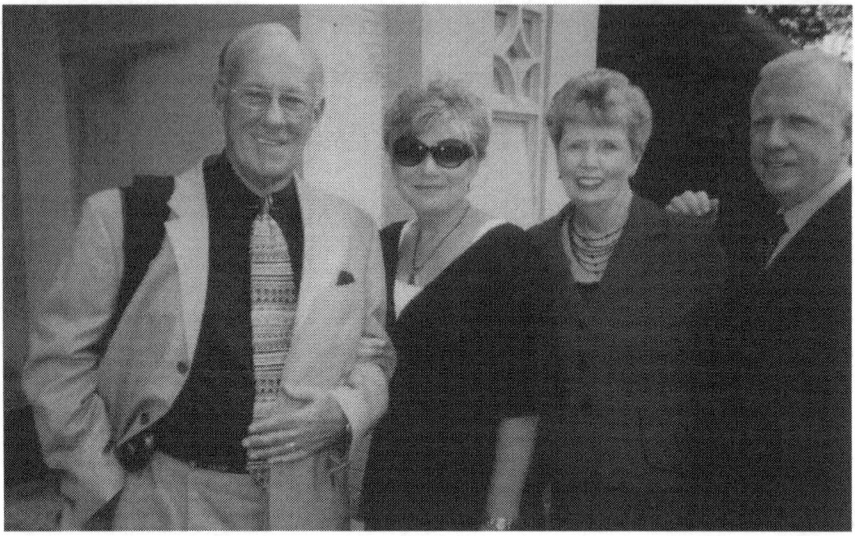

Me, Irene, my sister and brother outside church at my cousin's wedding in 2009. You can tell, can't you, that Irene couldn't wait to get on the dance floor. If she didn't have those glasses on, you'd see her smiling eyes, too.

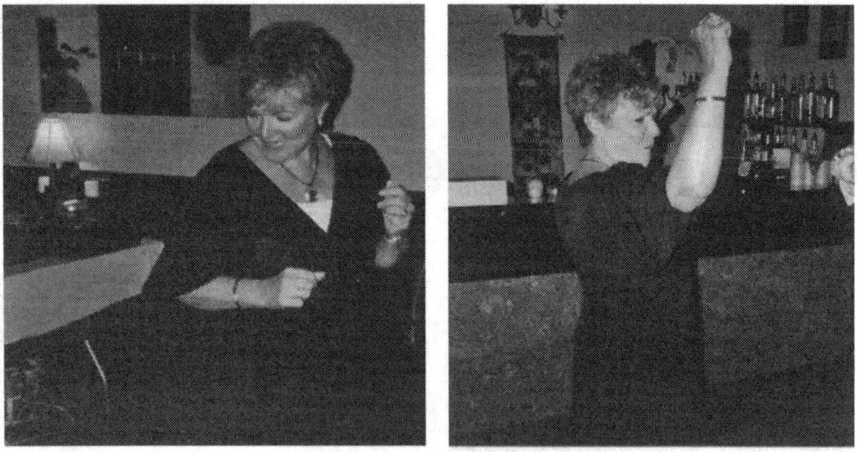

At my cousin's wedding, Irene was cutting up quite a rug. The wedding was in 2009 when Irene was six years into her cancer treatment. She was not going to let it stop her from experiencing her last few years on earth.

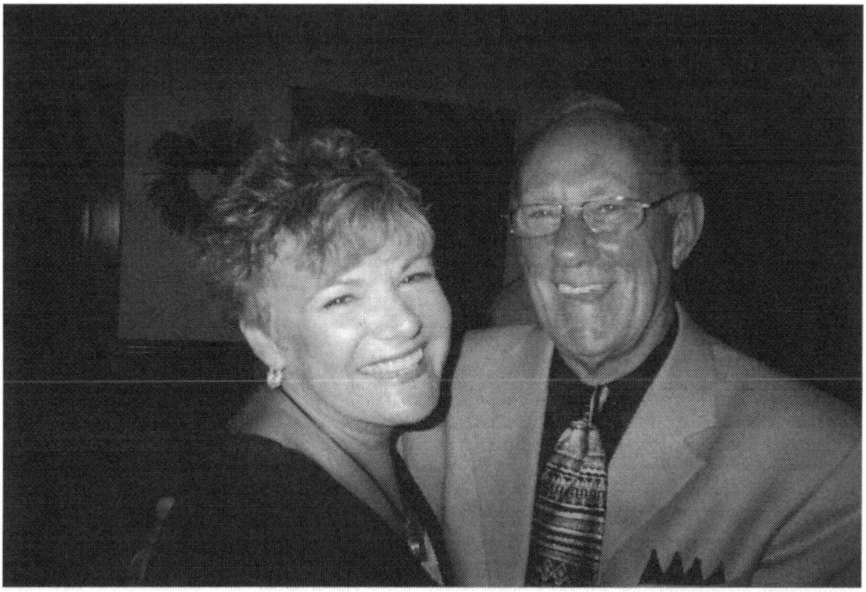

Always smiling in spite of her illness. After doing the Mummer's Strut (previous photos), Irene got me up to dance at my cousin's wedding, too.

I am very happy I was able to dance with her at that time. As fate would have it, that was our last public dance together.

In Loving Memory of

Irene Cooney

1/31/1953 – 6/22/2012

Funeral Mass:
11:00 AM
June 30, 2012
St. Thomas Aquinas Catholic Church
St. Cloud, Florida

OSCEOLA
MEMORY GARDENS
FUNERAL HOMES | CEMETERY | CREMATORY
SINCE 1958

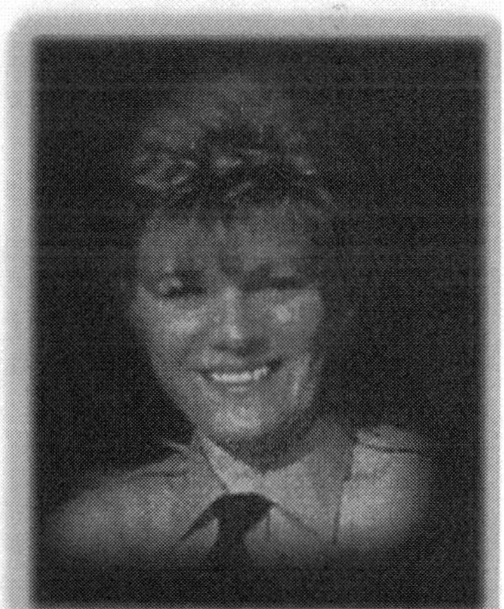

Chapter Seven

Riding the Rails

Irene wasn't up to plane rides or long drives. How about a train ride? Where to? Savannah, Georgia! Let's do it! It's about a five- or six-hour train ride with dining car and club car, like in the movies. Everyone should experience the intermingling in dining and club cars while traveling through the countryside. We visited Savannah before but only as a stopover, more or less. We decided to spend at least three or four days in that purely southern, very hospitable town.

Next step, after making the decision, was to contact my networking niece to arrange a great price at a great hotel. Done! I went to the train station and purchased the tickets. A few days later we were all packed and ready to go. Pat and Don drove us to the station and waited for the "All Aboard." It reminded me of the scene when Pat, my brother Mike, and my parents watched me board a train to San Antonio, Texas, to report for air force basic training many, many years before.

It also reminded me of the hobby I was involved in when I was recovering from cancer surgery. In the early '90s my sons played with the most elaborate HO gauge train platforms and setups that I built myself: switches galore, overpasses, underpasses and even HO gauge Philadelphia Transportation Company (PTC) trolley cars. I was a model train enthusiast at that time. And being interested in history, I studied railroads and how they helped create this nation. I knew all the various types of steam engines, from yard switchers to their diesel-electric successors that the Pennsylvania Railroad made famous among passengers and enthusiasts throughout the first half of the last century.

It was great therapy and an escape from my cancer diagnosis. It also nurtured the bonding between my sons and me.

Upon arrival in Savannah, Irene and I took a taxi from the train station directly to the hotel. I'll say it again—networking pays off. It was late so we decided to bed down and rise early to begin a full day. Savannah is picturesque and very Southern in character. We wanted to see it all in daytime.

The city is charming. Horse and carriage tours abound, as do bus and trolley rides, rolling passengers past every location of interest during jaunts of several hours. The unique antebellum architecture is as splendid as seen in the movies. As the carriage meandered slowly through the well-laid-out city, the trip was as leisurely and romantic as Irene and I could have hoped for. We stayed snuggled together, except every now and then, I jumped up to take pictures.

In the next few days, we ate at several very quaint restaurants and a couple of the best dining spots Savannah has to offer. The food was as good as it gets, and Irene handled the mini-vacation nicely. She smiled a lot. I always loved watching her taking in the sights. She was childlike as her eyes widened, and we passed by townhomes with very ornate ironwork on the wrap-around balconies. She would point to the railings and, wide-eyed, try to figure how long it would take to paint them.

"Oh, Tom! Look at that. That must be quite a job to repaint all that ironwork. My God! That railing goes all the way around both sides of the house too."

She was thinking about making it a project and probably disappointed that she had to leave the job at Home Depot. She could have bought the paint at an employee discount. She couldn't help herself.

Irene and I walked the river landing area that tourists must see when visiting Savannah. We heard that down by the river, St. Paddy's Day in March is as celebratory as any Irish bash in the country, including New York's or even Boston's famous parade and festivities. Our cares were distant as we strolled and munched on pralines in between meals.

I mentioned before that both Irene and I talk in our sleep. Mumbling is a more accurate way to describe it. The first time Irene brought it to my attention was when we stayed overnight in Charleston. It was my turn to tease her when she did it in Savannah.

After four days of gallivanting, we boarded the train again, looking forward to meeting any interesting personalities, such as we mingled with while in the dining car on our initial trip. We did meet new and very interesting people. Cancer was never discussed. My sister and brother-in-law picked us up at the train station. We were all smiles as we told them about our experiences in the grand old city of Savannah. Maybe the whole family could spend a few days there sometime in the future.

Back to Reality

08/05/2009: Back to chemo. Scan for restaging. One lesion in liver again. Starting chemo again. I'm getting Zantac and Benadryl first; then the cocktail.—I. C.

08/26/2009: Good response to FOLFIRI plus Avastin. 5-FU booster at home. Next appointment at clinic in four weeks for scan. Chemo in the meantime.—I. C.

09/23/2009: Continue FOLFIRI plus Avastin. Back at clinic in four weeks for scans, as usual.—I. C.

10/21/2009: Tumor Board said I'm not a candidate for radio-embolization right now (maybe later). They said the location of the lesion plus all the veins that grew in the area are problematic. There's another procedure they may use—RFA to the liver. They're giving me atropine and Benadryl again today before they give me the cocktail. I'm responding positively to my regular cocktail. Nighty-night.—I. C.

Radio-embolization (RE) for tumors in the liver is used when the lesion originated in or migrated to the liver, usually when surgery is not an immediate option because the tumor is too big and scattered or in a bad location. It's a very complicated procedure that requires access through main arteries supplying blood to the tumor.

During the procedure, tiny particles are sent through the bloodstream, lodge in the liver, and then emit pulses to kill or shrink the tumor. A small percentage of patients can suffer stomach ulcers and fistulas if the process doesn't go perfectly. It was very important to Irene's treatment agenda. All procedures were risky, but that was her life as a cancer patient.

As mentioned, radio frequency ablation (RFA) is a different procedure from RE and is used for many kinds of nodules, including liver. It, too, is used in both primary and metastatic lesions. It's the same basic process that I received for the potentially pre-cancerous cells at the bottom of my esophagus. Ablation uses high frequency to heat and, hopefully, destroy the dangerous cells. It can be an outpatient procedure because it is not as complicated or as dangerous as radio-embolization.

At that time, October 2009, the Tumor Board determined that Irene was not to be a candidate for the radio-embolization. Doctors, instead, considered RFA. She eventually did receive radio-embolization. And she was in that small percentage who had complications.

11/18/2009: Chemo today. Same as usual. FOLFIRI plus Avastin. Tom is here beside me, as usual.—I. C.

Irene's Mom Moves to Bradenton

I don't remember exactly when Maria moved to Bradenton, but I think it was during the holidays, late 2009 or early 2010. It was a time when both Irene and Maria needed more help. It was a big decision, but Maria was requiring a more watchful eye. She was becoming a little more forgetful, like me.

She was, by this time, in her mid-eighties. Her kitchen skills were not what they used to be. We had to be more cautious. We worried a little about leaving her alone. She needed medical attention on a more regular basis too. She should have been getting regular blood work. She had some health issues, and she needed dental work. She should have had more care than Irene and I could give her at that time.

Irene and I were very busy traveling to and from Moffitt, a three-hour round trip. Plus, we often spent seven hours or more at the hospital. Irene's hospital admissions were more frequent and were anticipated to be even more so. We were also trying to get the most out of the rest of

Irene's life. We could handle Maria's care up to this point, but there were almost a dozen of her adult family members over in Bradenton who could tend to her needs and did not have the schedule Irene and I were trying to maintain.

The family agreed that it was best if Maria moved to Bradenton so she was among her other, healthy children. Maria had two sons and a daughter there plus their spouses, and adult nephews and their partners. Maria's care could be shared among her family members in Bradenton to ensure she gets what is needed—a major concern of Irene's. And plenty of private and public organizations were available that the family could take advantage of to provide the required services.

In addition, it was getting a little more difficult for Irene and me to be bringing Maria to the west coast, considering how often we had doctor's appointments. Maria could not accompany us to the hospital during chemo sessions; the infusions lasted much too long. She would tire and want to go home. It was easier all around if Maria stayed in Bradenton and occasionally visited us, rather than the other way around. We kept her room available, however, whenever she wanted to stay over at our home.

12/02/2009: Continue chemo into the New Year with FOLFIRI and Avastin only. Lately, side effects have been bad. I've had about twelve infusions, I think, since I started it up again.—I. C.

12/16/2009: One last FOLFIRI and Avastin. I insisted on a break over the holidays. My feet and hands are on fire, and my mouth is very painful. Bad migraines. I'll pick it up again after Christmas when the side effects lessen. Will return after the holidays for evaluation.—I. C.

Medical History Summary through 2009

So far I've taken you through about six and a half years of Irene's illness and treatments. During that time, my contribution to Irene's care was accompanying her to all doctor and chemo appointments; being there before and after the surgeries to change some dressings; and administering daily shots of blood thinners and cell count boosters. On occasion, I rushed her to the local ER. I was a shoulder to cry on and generally, I did chores and provided comfort as much as possible.

During that time, when she felt up to it, Irene and I shopped together, traveled together, went to the movies together, enjoyed dinner and joined hands across the table, and visited relatives together. For the upcoming two and a half years, my caregiver role would expand. It was the same as before but included additional, more complex activities. Both of us grew more and more involved in her needs. There would be fewer treatment breaks in the future.

Bear in mind, we had many regular doctor visits throughout that whole time. There were appointments for periodic and diagnostic tests, including CAT, MRI, and PET scans, laboratory work, and numerous other routine and special tests, all during that entire period of treatment beginning in August 2003. Normally, when not on treatment break, doctors scanned at least once a month. Scans included the iodine injection or foul-tasting contrasts. Irene endured other intrusive procedures occasionally: rehydration, IV blood units, plus potassium and magnesium supplemental units delivered at the hospital through her port.

Many chemo sessions took place in between surgeries. We took breaks, but that mostly was during those periods in which no evidence of disease was detected, including during the immunotherapy study. There were many infusions following other surgeries. Irene had a couple of treatment breaks when she was just too weak and/or anemic. Several doctor-approved periods occurred when chemo was skipped or pushed forward a week or two to allow some normalcy in our lives, such as travel and mini-vacations.

I want to include a detailed medical history summary, 2003 through 2009, to give you a better idea of the cumulative impact and Irene's sufferings to this point, and so you can appreciate the strength and bravery that was required of her. The three years 2010, 2011, and 2012 were more intense than the first six and a half years.

2003: Feeling happier than ever after we became an item, we bought a home together when she returned from Florida. Irene began her long struggle with some abdominal pain. A colonoscopy, scans, and biopsies confirmed colon cancer that also metastasized to her liver. She was scheduled right away for surgery on August 29, 2003, at Nazareth

Hospital in Philadelphia. About eighteen inches of her colon was removed, along with twelve lymph nodes, seven of which were diseased.

The tumor in her colon was tennis-ball sized. The surgeon could not remove the lesion in her liver. She spent two weeks in recovery enduring that annoying nasal-gastro tube and all the other inconveniences associated with a hospital stay. While in the hospital, she threw a blood clot in her right lung, which extended her stay a bit longer and required the start of lifelong blood thinner injections at home. After her discharge, we arranged chemotherapy sessions at Fox Chase Cancer Center, also in Philadelphia.

After recovery from the colon resection, her port was inserted in her left upper chest in readiness for the upcoming infusions. The placement was a little complicated surgically but ultimately successful. She received several chemo sessions and was readied for liver surgery the following December. I'll refer you to that list of side effects to get an idea of what Irene was going through after she started chemo. At that time, the nausea and hair loss bothered her the most, but she soon realized that would be the least of her worries.

The surgeon removed the right lobe of her liver on December 16, 2003, and also installed a portable device, an arterial pump, that dispensed chemo (same side effects) twenty-four hours a day, seven days a week. A week in the hospital included that irritating NG tube and the new appendage (the pump), which was refilled monthly with her cocktail. Her doctor accommodated us now and then by removing it so we could travel more conveniently. Irene wore that bag intermittently for many months.

All the above occurred and concluded in the span of four months at the close of 2003.

2004: Two months after liver surgery, in February 2004, I rushed Irene to the ER at Jeanes Hospital, next door to FCCC. Her right leg was swollen. The diagnostic scan determined she had another dangerous blood clot. That was two so far. The medical team concluded, as cancer patients are more prone to throw blood clots, that Irene should have a Greenfield filter placed in her right femoral artery. They hoped to prevent future clots from traveling through her system to her heart. That could kill her. As you can imagine, stress was building in our lives. Within a week, Irene had the mappings and scans required and then underwent yet another sedation and procedure for the filter placement.

In the meantime, Irene still received intermittent infusions, mostly on a weekly basis. On March 3, 2004, exactly one year after she was reinstated to the PPD, she was notified she was number one on the detective promotional list. She was to report to the police academy for detective training. She had to decline that coveted position. That was a great disappointment to Irene, as you might imagine. She was deeply hurt, and she quietly wept but accepted her fate.

In April 2004, Irene had an unsuccessful procedure to remove the Greenfield filter. In addition, since the start of the year, she had about a dozen to fifteen additional intermittent infusions. It turned out to be a good thing that the filter was enmeshed with new vascular routes and couldn't be removed. Irene threw more clots in the future. She also had a clear mammogram in April.

Remember, Irene was managing, with both difficulty and support, to go to work, despite nausea, fatigue, pimples, rashes, mucositis, fissures, sore feet and hands, multiple visits to the hospital, and other side effects resulting from her continued infusions and the chemo drip from the external pump. She always smiled at work, I'm told.

She finally felt some relief later when we got a treatment break. The constant scans revealed no hypermetabolic activity. We traveled often. She would still have the external pouch, though. Then, in late summer, along came those hurricanes and the added concern she had for my well-being.

The external pump was finally removed on October 15, with just a little bit of a problem. The connector-lead imbedded in her liver had to be left in place. The surgeon brought her back twice for scans to make sure blood and air that accumulated during the procedure had dissipated and drained. That debris was painful for a while.

During 2004, Irene had at least nine blood draws, an equal number of various scans, her second blood clot, placement of the Greenfield, and the unsuccessful attempt to remove it. Since beginning chemotherapy, not counting the twenty-four-hour drip via the pump, Irene endured the tough side effects of about forty infusions. She had a well-deserved treatment break at the end of 2004. We had an enjoyable holiday season.

2005: By March 21, 2005, a PET scan showed new small lesions on Irene's liver, spleen, right lower lung, and an abdominal lymph node. The following month, she restarted weekly chemo sessions at FCCC, trying to get at those new nodules. Several pretty bad side effects lasted for months. The oncologist reduced the dose a little because of her previous severe reactions.

We both had heart scans at the University of Pennsylvania Hospital, which were offered to active and retired police. I was in great shape; Irene's heart was perfect. Nothing else to do except get married.

Even though the dosage was reduced, the side effects were more severe than usual. We couldn't do any traveling. She worked just about every day, even though she felt nauseated all the time. She still wore her smile. Nobody knew how much she was suffering.

In September, when previous scans were compared, a new scan revealed no evidence of disease on Irene's liver, spleen, or abdominal lymph node, but the PET scan showed a small lesion in her lower right lung. That's where the original blood clot formed. Evidently, the chemo sessions she started in the spring were doing the job. She was clear, except for the lung nodule. Miraculous!

Then the October scan, when compared to the previous month, showed no change. The lung nodule, still a concern, did not enlarge and nothing else was showing up. She continued the weekly chemo sessions until she asked for a break over the holidays, which she received. The team was happy to reward her. She had nearly thirty-five additional infusions during 2005. That brought the total to about seventy-five thus far in her treatment.

2006: The scans in January 2006 showed that the lung nodule was slightly increased, which created more angst in our lives. The node was still small, though. Irene needed the holiday break to continue longer. Even after the previous treatment break, she was worn down by the multiple side effects she suffered. The doctors agreed the added time would build her up for possible lung surgery in a few months. The nodule's rate of growth allowed a respite. It was worth the risk for a couple more months of feeling normal and regaining strength. She still went to work regularly. This break would be the longest one she had so far.

In April 2006, the lung nodule showed another enlarging. A biopsy proved it metastasized from the colon. There was a nodule on an adrenal gland too. That was devastating to us. Irene and I both shed a tear over that news. It was an emotional roller coaster.

Scans in May revealed the lung nodule was still there, but the one on the adrenal gland was not detected. Chemo restarted right away. The side effects returned immediately. Irene endured more discomfort and suffering.

The scan in late May showed that the nodule in her lung wasn't responding as well as desired. She suffered a few more chemos during May and June, and then they were stopped. She readied for another surgery on June 28. On the 20th, we made all the arrangements with the surgeon. That surgery was very successful. Irene retired from the PPD in July. We moved to Florida.

The new oncologist at Moffitt Cancer Center in Tampa, Florida, advised Irene to continue maintenance chemo. Irene had two chemo sessions locally and, disappointed in the service, we decided to travel the three-hour round trip to Tampa for her infusions.

She started infusions at Tampa in late July 2006, and they continued on a biweekly basis until October, when scans were repeated. By Halloween, there was no evidence of disease on the scans! No metabolic activity was detected! Irene negotiated another treatment break. The break carried us into and beyond the holidays.

Irene had lung surgery and nearly a dozen infusions over the past six or seven months. Long-term chemo really wears a patient down. As the number of infusions increases, so does the resultant debilitation. Irene now had had about eighty-seven sessions. She was less than three and a half years into her treatment and already had several surgeries and other procedures in addition to those chemo sessions. But at this time she was beating the odds.

2007: In January 2007, a small lesion showed up in the left lobe of the liver, but there was nothing in the lung. She had another chemo session (eighty-eight) that had horrid side effects. She couldn't get out of bed. It was discontinued, and we started talks about surgery again. Within three weeks, on February 12, 2007, she went under the knife once more, after all the thorough pre-admission diagnostic testing.

Other than not feeling well, Irene participated fully in agreeing to have the surgery on the left lobe of her liver. The scans determined that the node was near the surface and accessible, so they would be able to go inside through an incision and wedge out the tumor. They didn't have to remove the entire lobe. They'd taken the entire right lobe of the liver last time.

During the operation, the surgeon also removed part of Irene's intestines near the stomach and also incised other spots in the area, resulting in a slight kink in the small intestine exiting the stomach. That threatened to interrupt digestion. It turned out okay for the time being. She could eat a little bit before she was discharged. She spent six days in the hospital that time.

So, 2007 started off with severe nausea, diarrhea, and other side effects. By February 12, the liver/stomach surgery, including Irene's six-day hospital stay, kept us on edge. She restarted chemo, adding about six more, bringing her total to ninety-four.

By May, no hypermetabolic activity was detected. Let *me* say it this time: whoopee! That qualified Irene for an immunotherapy study. Irene had the preparatory and painful femoral artery invasion, leukapheresis, by the physician's assistant who caused her to scream in pain. Tissue and blood work was forwarded to Duke University, where they concocted a serum.

Once started, the study lasted four months, with regular visits to the clinic for tests and injections. Irene didn't have any chemo sessions during this time, just injections. That period was a relief but ended in disappointment. The lesions returned. Hope was there and then was dashed.

Biweekly chemo sessions began again by fall. After the infusion at the hospital, Irene came home with a bag containing 5-FU attached to her port. It infused over forty-six hours and then a home health nurse visited to detach it. The nurse drew blood and submitted it for examination. Four chemo sessions followed by the end of the year, bringing the total to ninety-eight, not counting the home infusions each time. We also drove to numerous visits and diagnostic tests during that time.

2008: By January 2008, Irene had a recurrence in her liver. She was infused with a cocktail that gave her a reaction that was too severe. She agreed to it, even though she knew the effects were terrible. Finally, the doctors switched her to one that turned out to be less effective in the long run, because in January 2009, a year later, the nodule reappeared.

To give Irene periodic rests, we took a few treatment breaks by occasionally taking three weeks instead of two between infusions. The staging scans and blood work continued through the end of the year. By the end of 2008, Irene added approximately twenty sessions, bringing the total to 118, conservatively speaking.

In December 2008, Irene suffered very severe pain, diarrhea, fever, and blood in her stool. She was dehydrated and anemic, too. I rushed her to the local ER. She was admitted and spent four very uncomfortable days in a hospital bed. She was discharged just in time for the holidays, diagnosis unknown.

2009: The year 2009 was like 2008. As mentioned, it started off with a recurrence of the liver nodule. Chemo was restarted right away. She couldn't get out of bed for several days after each session. There was metabolic activity near her right lung. She refused to stop chemo at this time, saying she wanted this disease "out of my body." Irene had to be wheeled to the infusion room because she was so weak. She received that session in one of the "penthouses." Nine or ten more chemo sessions brought the total to around 127, conservatively speaking.

During this period, at home, after each infusion at Moffitt, the visiting nurse removed the 5-FU dispenser bag, drew blood, and flushed the port lead. I injected the blood thinner shots twenty-four hours after the portable bag removal. The pain in Irene's stomach was very sharp, and Irene's hair was falling out again.

Chemotherapy by August included Avastin. FOLFIRI plus Avastin continued through December. Irene suffered serious side effects, and the liver tumor still increased in size.

In December, after diagnostic scans, the FOLFIRI part of the cocktail was stopped because it was not effective anymore, in addition to the side effects being too debilitating for Irene. She continued to be infused with Avastin only. Irene needed a rest over the holidays. The oncologist gave her a two-month break to recuperate.

A positive decision by the Tumor Board, however, opened the pathway to try radio-embolization—theraspheres. It had recently been approved for colon cancer if metastasis was only to the liver and not more widespread. We scheduled the procedure for the spring of 2010, after extensive preparatory mapping exams and tests.

Before I describe the years of 2010, 2011, and 2012, please keep in mind the pain and discomfort that Irene braved as you read the description of her battle and the extraordinary stamina required to deal with her situation. Most people who receive chemotherapy probably don't receive anywhere near the number of lengthy infusions that Irene did. I don't know the record, but Irene is surely in the running for the most ever. Consider all those associated side effects, too, including the emotional ones.

I noticed Irene was gradually weakening. Sitting on the lanai watching a diving water fowl surface with a little fish in its beak, I reminded her that the Tumor Board had approved her for radio-embolization.

"Tom, I'm getting really tired. Do you think this new procedure will work?"

"Yes, honey. Think about it when it does work. This could be the end of your cancer if they're able to destroy that one last nodule in the liver. The doctors are even excited for you. The chances are in our favor. We could have many more years together. It'll be a good time for us, honey, free of this disease. It could release us to be finally done with chemos, scans, and the whole world we've been living in. We could have the longest treatment break ever."

Irene reached for me from her lounge chair to mine with her arms extended. She beckoned with her hands. "Please gimme a big hug, handsome. I hope and pray you're right."

"Don't worry, honey. We're together."

"I love you, Tom."

2010: Radio-Embolization

In late December 2009, the doctors discontinued 5-FU and irinotecan (FOLFIRI) and during January 2010 continued regular infusions of Avastin only. That brought her total to about 138 chemotherapies by the end of the month. The chemo was working. Only the liver nodule was active.

02/02/2010: Whoopee! Latest scans didn't detect any other lesions except in my liver.—I. C.

Scans at this point revealed her cancer was progressing only in the left lobe of her liver. That was remarkable *quantity* of life extension, in and of itself, after six and a half years of aggressive therapy. Irene was way out ahead of the odds. It was a relatively good thing that only her liver tumor was active.

But by early February, she still had terrible pain in her hands and feet, along with very troublesome mouth sores. She couldn't eat, walk, or use her hands in a normal manner. By mid-February, she felt increasing pain in the right upper quadrant of her abdomen also.

Our medical team got together and finally convinced the Tumor Board to approve specific targeting of the liver lesion with radio-embolization. Irene was re-evaluated to see if that lead left over from that exterior arterial pump might interfere with the procedure. That lead had been there since way back in December 2003.

The board decided the lead would not interfere with the high-tech procedure. If this regimen worked, it would be miraculous—six and a half years already achieved after a diagnosis of fourth stage cancer and then a possibility of even greater extension of Irene's life.

In radio-embolization, a beam of tiny beads, or spheres, directly target the lesion with the hope of destroying it. The "gun" is inserted and guided inside the patient through the femoral artery system. It is not radiation. The theraspheres have direct contact with the tumor. They bombard it.

After signing the obligatory consent forms, the procedure went forward. First, a few preparatory tests were needed before the actual radio-embolization. Irene's insides had to be completely mapped as a precaution against leakage of the beads into other areas surrounding her liver. If any pathways were detected, they had to be clamped off.

To send the mapping dye into her abdomen, a probe was inserted into her femoral artery. After anesthetizing Irene, these experts were able to thread the catheter up her right femoral to the area and then into her liver. (That area of her lower abdomen was very vascular, remember.) Analysis of Irene's abdomen revealed no extraordinary problems. They found no reason preventing the radio-embolization. This could actually be the end of Irene's suffering after all these years, if the procedure was successful. Or it could be the beginning of a cascade of problems.

03/02/2010: After preparatory CAT scans, doctors performed an image-guided liver angiogram to map the lesion in the left lobe of my liver. They targeted the liver tumor and believed they got it. After the procedure they inserted a seal at the right femoral where the catheter entered. There were no guarantees regarding the procedure.—I. C.

In the meantime, chemotherapy was restarted. She completed two additional chemos (total: 140) while we waited for follow-up scans to measure the results of the radio-embolization.

We felt good about the positive effect this "star wars" therapy might produce. It could extend her life significantly. At first, hopes were high that the effort would be successful in reducing or eliminating the sole remaining lesion in her liver. When she was released from the hospital, she ate a little bit. That pleasure was one that she hadn't fully appreciated in the recent past. But that pleasure soon ended. She had lost quite a bit of weight. Irene and I anxiously anticipated a return to the hospital for scans to compare baseline diagnostic tests to find out if we could celebrate success.

But while at home for a few weeks, Irene's abdominal pain increased to a level that was unbearable, even for Irene. Something was seriously wrong. We made arrangements to have the medical team diagnose the problem. An endoscopy was necessary.

03/23/2010: Disappointment again! The procedure caused two holes to form in my stomach near where the liver/stomach surgery of February 12, 2007, had occurred at Moffitt. The fistulas are like ulcers and cause pain, discomfort, and vomiting when I would try to eat. I was basically unable to eat at that time. Total parenteral nutrition (TPN) feeding at home through my port would probably be necessary.—I. C.

Unfortunately, there was a complication with the radio-embolization procedure that resulted in a sea change in Irene's troubles. Two large holes formed in Irene's stomach. This setback was momentous.

Medically, the holes were termed gastro/hepatic (stomach/liver) fistulas. The holes were created in the wall of Irene's stomach. They were not the usual type of ulcers, such as open sores. They were more like raw holes. The stomach fistulas formed a tunnel. Picture a flexible tube, less than an inch in diameter, bent so that both circular and symmetrical open ends are seen—that's an idea of what was observed in the endoscopic procedure that discovered them.

It took several days for the theraspheres to create that pathway. Normally, if such an opening occurred in someone's stomach, contents would leak into the abdomen, causing a life-threatening condition (e.g., peritonitis) within a short time. In Irene's case, her liver sealed off that escape. The fistulas were blocked by her liver pressing up against them.

In Irene's medical records, I have the endoscopic photos of the fistulas. It was obvious the holes were caused by a penetrating burn that just seared its way from one end to the other, like bullet holes. They are ugly: red, raw, and black where more severe burning took place. I can only imagine the pain Irene felt. Once the theraspheres started creating that path, nothing could stop them, and there was no way to control those little beads. We had to hope they ran their course and that the resultant damage would heal by Irene's body's recuperative powers alone. The doctors had not seen this situation before.

It became obvious after a while that Irene's condition required most of her nutrition to be delivered externally—total parenteral nutrition (TPN). This was new to both of us and involved something we did not anticipate. Irene's nutrition now depended on external, unnatural means.

In the meantime, still in pain, Irene had two more chemo sessions, bringing the total to about 142. It was suspected the chemo might be interfering with the healing of the fistulas, so it was discontinued again, while the medical team made the arrangements for TPN. After several interviews with the nutritionist, and consults with Moffitt's pharmacy, conversations with suppliers and home health agencies who delivered in our area, the team estimated the first shipment would arrive at our home in early May.

We continued to wait and hope that after a period on TPN, Irene would be able to experience the pleasure of eating orally again. In the meantime, Irene took a deserved treatment break. During our wait, Irene was prescribed two powerful medications to speed up the healing of the fistulas and decrease her discomfort. We added them to the long list of her regular medications. Thankfully, the prescriptions did help. The pain eased a bit.

03/30/2010: Scans show fistulas might be stabilizing. Still can't eat much. It was decided that when TPN starts, Tom will do it at home. Nurse will come to our home and instruct Tom. I'll probably start TPN in early May after arrangements are made. Nothing to do but wait.—I. C.

After verification of the diagnosis, the TPN process was put into motion. We just waited for the design of the best menu for Irene. The team was deciding which medical supply company serving our area would deliver to us and of course on insurance company approval.

Ireland, Germany, and a Volcanic Eruption

My youngest son went back to school for his RN degree. (He has continued toward his advanced degrees since then, I'm happy to say; it pleased Irene greatly. She encouraged him to go further.) Irene suggested that Chris be rewarded with a trip to Ireland and Germany. I told you Irene was generous and that she adored my sons. She said it would be a good time for me, too, to take advantage of the current lull and treatment break and go with Chris—the bonding thing, you know!

Irene was unable to travel, but she and I were just sitting and waiting at this point. She eased my concern a little by saying she could spend time between home and her sister's in Bradenton. She could visit with Maria. That would be a respite for Irene. My sister and family were also close by and available, just in case Irene needed anything. Irene was still driving at the time, too.

She wanted to make it a gift for Chris and me. He, very thankfully, enthusiastically supported the idea. I resisted, but Irene insisted. Chemo had stopped—it wasn't as effective as desired—and she wasn't feeling really bad (at least that's what she said). And we were just waiting for the TPN recipe and program to be completed. We had a few weeks, until early May.

I made the arrangements. Chris and I took off for Europe. The plan was to spend four days driving north up the west coast of Ireland and then across the midlands down to Dublin for a few days. From Dublin, we'd fly to Berlin, spend a couple days, and drive south toward Munich. We scheduled a return to Ireland from Germany and then would motor along the southern coast of Ireland. The trip would be about twelve days total, door to door. We began our journey in early April. TPN was expected to start in early May. I constantly called Irene, who said everything was fine at home but that Dusty, our cat, missed me. She told us to enjoy ourselves.

We planned to visit the family farm in Hattenhofen, Germany, where Irene's parents worked during WWII. We had no idea if the farm or the farmer even existed anymore. We figured that would be "verrrry interesting," as that character in *Hogan's Heroes* and *Saturday Night Live* used to say. After a torturous drive up a cart path, we found the wife of the son of the farmer for whom Irene's parents had worked. Unbelievable, but true! We took pictures and videos. (Later, Maria was excited when she saw them.)

But then on April 14, a volcano erupted in Iceland, and air travel all over Europe was canceled. Irene called me, frantic that Chris and I might be injured and breathing volcanic ash. She said the news media made it sound as if hundreds were dying. We knew nothing—like Sergeant Schultz in *Hogan's Heroes*. So naturally, if we were near death, we'd better tune in. We watched the news. All flights in and out of Europe were grounded.

We were marooned in Bavaria, Germany—not a bad place to be stuck. Our only worry was to be home in time for Irene's TPN and Chris's next semester. We drove north from Munich and found a little town where the rates hadn't skyrocketed. We settled in for the next week.

When we finally got a flight out of Munich, we flew straight to the United States. We missed the second leg of our Ireland tour. Next time!

We were happy to get home. We returned in plenty of time for Irene's TPN sessions. Chris's brother, Tommy, picked him up at Newark Airport. After a relatively short delay, I got a flight to Orlando. Irene picked me up. I really missed her during that trip. By April 21, thirteen days after Chris and I left the States, I was happy to be back at home with Irene.

"I love you, Irene."

"I love you, too, Tom. Glad you're home. Gimme a big hug and kiss, handsome."

We both missed each other—a lot!

Total Parenteral Nutrition (TPN)

When my son and I returned from Europe, Irene and I waited patiently for the medical team to arrange for the equipment and the nutrient prescription to be delivered to our home. In the meantime, Irene wasn't able to eat much because of those two holes that were burned into her stomach. When she tried, eating caused pain, and she regurgitated. She was losing weight in addition to being very uncomfortable.

I needed to become even more involved in Irene's care. TPN is often given in a hospital setting, but we wanted Irene to remain at home. I preferred to administer the necessary nutrition rather than a visiting nurse. So did Irene. All I needed was some instruction.

Irene, the medical team, and our families understood that my involvement kept and extended the personal attachment between Irene and me as a caregiver. I would have felt like a bystander if someone else did it if I was able. Irene showed her appreciation when everyone agreed it was well within my capabilities. It was not rocket science. She always trusted me completely and showed it with her big smiles. I had hoped for that.

04/28/2010: Restarted chemo. Irinotecan and Erbitux again. It worked in the past.—I. C.

04/30/2010: Another hospital admission. Tom called Direct Referral and arranged for me to be admitted back into the hospital (Moffitt). Severe pain in my abdomen. Another endoscopy to check on healing of the ulcers. Some improvement, but it still hurts.—I. C.

Irene was still in the hospital when, on May 1, 2010, I went home to take care of Dusty and found the TPN delivery at the front door, packed with refrigerant. I wondered how long it had been there, but it still felt cold. There were bags marked "2000 milliliter" (2 liters), and also contained gloves, tape, syringes, telescoping pole, and a lot of little medicine vials. I put it all in the spare fridge. We were going to have to get used to this.

05/04/2010: Had some infection. Meds in hospital helped. Discharged. Tom will set up all the TPN paraphernalia and add the meds to the nutrition after he mixes it all up. We'll practice because Tom will be going to Tommy and Irene's wedding in a little over a month. I have to get good at it.—I. C.

In many cases, there's no reason for someone to be hospitalized during long-term TPN, if a family member does it. Home health nurses are used often today also. Visiting nurses are professional, of course, but you may have different nurses every day, a few of whom may not care as much as others. Keep in mind the emotional impact this setup has because of not being able to feed oneself. This measure was a tremendous loss of independence for someone like Irene (or for anyone). Irene needed to know she was loved. I wanted her to know I would do whatever it took to make the process as comfortable as possible for her.

You can do it, too. Your loved one will appreciate it. Your bonding will become even greater. It's very personal. You'll see it in his or her smiling eyes. In a short time, you'll be eager to do it. It becomes effortless for you, because you are helping the one you love.

You just have to put aside any fear or trepidation you may feel. You are doing it because you love her. When the love is as deep as some profess, you overcome any difficulties, whether they are travel, chores you can do later, or any other interruption of your normal schedule. We would die for those we love deeply, and we wouldn't have a fear of doing it. The challenge is to ask yourself: "Do I love this person enough to put aside any inconvenience and give of my time?"

Anyone with the desire to do it should not have any difficulty in administering TPN at home after some initial guidance by a visiting nurse. I watched many years of Irene's external sustenance during Irene's many hospital stays.

I saw all the little preparatory steps: masks; gloves; alcohol swabs; inserting lines into the hanging containers and ensuring there were no air bubbles; using the additional "Y" junction in the main lines to add antibiotics, vitamins, or painkillers periodically, without having to detach the main access; adjusting flow rates, either on calibrated pumps or by eye, with that little drip-controlling thumb wheel in the main lines; and several other routine movements that attending nurses go through during the process of delivering TPN and medications.

Nurses accomplish many activities that I am certainly not qualified to perform. Administering TPN is *not* one of them. There's more to it than what I just mentioned, of course.

The TPN menu is very specific to the nutritional needs of each patient. A medical team consisting of the attending doctor, nutritionist, dietician, pharmacist, supplier, and (when regular blood draws are needed) a visiting nurse. The team considers a patient's age, gender, height, weight, and type of illness in designing the proper milliliters/grams of each and every ingredient.

In Irene's case, the two-liter bag minimally contained fats, sugars, and amino acids, plus minerals that everyone needs for basic nutrition. For example, out of Irene's daily prescribed dose total of 1,820 milliliters, there were 250 milliliters of fats in her menu. There were eleven other components, each with precise percentages relative to the 1,820 ml total volume. Vitamins, other minerals, and antibiotics can be added or subtracted. At one point, lipids were reduced in Irene's menu to reduce constipation. TPN has its own peculiar side effects. Constipation was a relief for Irene to an extent—she'd had diarrhea for so long—but we all must evacuate, or we become impacted. That's very dangerous. Constipation can contribute to diverticulitis, among other ailments.

We received a special delivery of a week's supply each week in refrigerated packaging. The supplier usually called before and after delivery to ensure everything was in good order. After inspecting it all for correct prescription, leaks, or spoilage, I placed it all in our spare refrigerator, along with the accompanying antibiotics, minerals, and vitamins. In addition to all those basic lifeline ingredients, Irene was prescribed two antibiotics and two additional mineral supplements: potassium and magnesium.

During our first session at home, I took notes. A visiting nurse went through each step of delivering the TPN, emphasizing clean versus sterile. Nothing can touch the floor. If I picked up any item from the floor, I had to wash my hands again and put on new gloves. Visitors also had to be made aware of the importance of protecting Irene from the risk of infection. Even our cat had to know not to get too close. That was tough for Irene and for Dusty. She used to love to kiss our Dusty in the past.

Everything came in sterile packaging: syringes for flushing the port and its lead, syringes containing saline and heparin (a blood thinner plus a clog preventer), gloves, masks, flow lines, connectors to access Irene's port, adhesive tape, the hanging pole, Sharp's biohazard disposal container—everything that was needed.

All was provided and delivered in sufficient amounts, arranged by Moffitt's registered nutritionist, the supplier's team, and registered pharmacist. The supplier also provided a how-to booklet and pamphlets describing the entire process, including tips on leaks, travel, and any emergency. I could always refer to it, if necessary. The supplier and nurses could be contacted 24/7, just in case.

When I was ready to connect Irene to the nutrients, I extended and arranged the wheeled pole on which the two-liter bag, containing all the fluids, hangs. I allowed everything to get to room temperature, about an hour. Initially, the main bag of nutrients was clamped, separating the top half, containing a clear solution, from the bottom half, containing a milky solution. The bottom had most of the suspended nutrients (lipids, for example). When ready to begin the process, I removed the clamp and massaged the top and bottom ingredients together, mixing them thoroughly. They had to be mixed shortly before administering them. The mixture couldn't just lay around.

The additive antibiotics and mineral supplements came individually in vials. I removed the protective cap from the little vials and sterilized the rubber sealer tops of the vials with a swab, so I could safely puncture the rubber and withdraw the meds into the syringe. There is a knack to both preparing a syringe (clearing a vacuum) and then actually withdrawing solutions into the syringe. The nurse showed me how to "pop" the vacuum. I was familiar with getting rid of any air inside the gradated syringe. I did it many times. You simply release just a tiny drop of the fluid after withdrawing it from the vial. You've seen it done a thousand times. Don't squirt yourself or your loved one in the face if you ever do it.

I was told to use separate syringes for each of the two antibiotics. For the two mineral supplements, I used the same syringe to withdraw those, as they can be mixed with each other without risk of contamination. After swabbing a one-way access valve at the top of that big main bag I'd previously massaged, I then injected the antibiotics and supplements separately into that access valve. I massaged it all again, got rid of the used syringes and vials appropriately, and hung the big bag on the pole. It wasn't to be hung too high; it might be top-heavy and difficult to move around safely without toppling it. It also wasn't to be so low that the feed had to fight gravity, either.

So, the nutrients were prepared and then had to be delivered into Irene's system through her port. The TPN was to flow and provide Irene with nutrition within an hour or so after bringing it to room temperature. I couldn't leave the concoction sitting around too long. The five-foot-long see-through flexible main delivery line accessed the goodies bag via a second valve at its bottom. The line had a connector at one end to access the bag and another connector at its other end that fit onto the lead coming out of Irene's port. It had a tiny thumb-adjustable wheel inline to open, close, and control the nutrition flow rate.

I pushed the main line connector into the bag at that second valve's receptor up to its hilt. I just had to be sure I closed the inline thumb-control flow adjuster or I'd make a mess. That valve was the doorway for the fluid to flow through the main line. Sterility was important. I had to be careful not to let the main line touch the floor.

A visiting nurse, by law and insurance regulations, still had to come to the house once a week to change Irene's port lead and take blood samples for analysis. Remember, the port was under Irene's skin and made a connection to her bloodstream inside her chest. An RN had to make that access invasion each time. It stayed in place during the week to allow me to make Irene's daily connection.

When not in use, her port was unattached to the outside world, but a lead was necessary to connect Irene's port to the supply of nutrients and chemo. That lead had a needle with a length and diameter exactly correct for Irene's port on one end and an external connector on the other. It also had a "Y" junction at the end so meds could be delivered while the main line was connected to various sources, such as TPN, chemo, and fluids.

The lead was about six to eight inches long. A nurse knew exactly where to puncture Irene's skin in order to insert the needle perfectly in the middle, so that the vein to which the port was sewn was accessed. Too far, too shallow, or too much to the right or left, and Irene's bloodstream would be missed. That's why it took an *experienced* nurse to do it, not just *any* nurse.

Once accessed, the lead became the gateway to Irene's bloodstream. That lead, with the needle inserted into Irene's veins, was what had to be changed weekly by a visiting nurse. When Irene received each infusion at the hospital, the lead was always removed so it didn't interfere with Irene's clothing in between weekly sessions. During TPN, however, the lead hanging out of her port was a continuing appendage taped to her chest and readily available to me for each daily administration of the nutrients on weekdays.

So, after flushing Irene's port through the lead that a nurse changed weekly and clearing any air bubbles in the main line from the big bag, I attached the five-foot-long main line that I changed at least daily, always flushing, to her port lead's connector. I opened the flow and eyeballed the number of drips per minute flowing into that see-through cylindrical drip measurer that nurses are always intently peering at.

In our case, Irene was to initially receive nutrition over fifteen hours, from 4:00 PM to 7:00 AM. It usually lasted longer for one reason or another. She was attached to the wheeled pole most of that time. I could always detach her and close the line for brief periods to give her some relief, as long as I flushed afterward and again before reattaching the main line to get the flow going again.

At first, Irene received 1,820 ml over fifteen hours, as she wasn't able to eat anything by mouth. As time went by and the fistulas were healing, Irene became more able to supplement the TPN with eating.

The volume of nutrients was incrementally reduced to about 1,250 ml per session.

Ideally, the nutrients were to flow at a slower rate during the first and last couple hours during each session. After a few hours, I could get a good idea of any adjustments to the rate of flow that was required. We closely watched the fluid level in the gradated see-through bag to ensure constant flow. I would also disconnect and flush with syringes of saline solution every four hours or so to guard against clogging due to kinks in the flexible line while we slept.

When the hanging bag emptied by the end of the session, I just detached and discarded everything appropriately and finished up with a flush of her port with saline and a premeasured amount of heparin, the blood thinner and clog preventer.

Later, when Irene had a feeding tube surgically implanted into her abdomen, we had a pump that regulated the flow through the tube. But for the TPN, I depended on the thumb control to increase or decrease the volume of nutrients entering Irene's body through her port.

One last note: the medical field is full of acronyms. In order to easily remember the flushing process and administering of any meds directly, someone originated SASH: *S*aline; *A*dminister medications; *S*aline; *H*eparin. Each and every time I connected and disconnected Irene, I would go through the SASH steps.

Irene and I gradually got used to the whole process. She pulled and pushed the pole around the house and to the bathroom all the time during the period she was on TPN.

I hope the foregoing description is sufficient to encourage you to administer TPN yourself, after instruction and guidance by a medical professional.

Irene always made light of her situation.

"That meal tasted better than the last one, Tom," she'd tease. "Did you use some extra seasoning?"

Or she'd say, "Tom, please put some fruit in my feed bag today."

"Sure, honey. Just close your eyes. It'll be blueberries today. You love blueberries. So does your mom. Okay. It's flowing, honey."

"Mmm, mmm. Tastes great! You're so good to me, Tommy."

Chapter Eight

Hospital Admission—Again

Our routine continued normally for a few weeks. We drove to Moffitt Cancer Center in the morning to get biweekly chemo (total of 146 by June 10, 2010). Once home in the afternoon, I attached the TPN.

A little over a month after being discharged from the hospital, however, Irene was admitted again.

06/10/2010: Hospital admission! Went to a regular visit to GI clinic at Moffitt for chemo but I was feeling low with symptoms of weakness, diarrhea, vomiting, fatigue (which may be associated with stomach fistulas). Doctors hospitalized me. They took regular CAT scans to determine the healing progress of the fistulas. Healing is anticipated to be a very slow process because of the therasphere beads. After a few days in the hospital, there were signs of a fungus on my tongue, too, like before. Total parenteral nutrition (TPN) plus antifungal and antibiotics through my port were prescribed in the hospital, and Tom will continue them at home when I get discharged next week.—I. C.

A PET scan during her hospital stay in mid-June revealed that same stubborn hypermetabolic nodule in Irene's liver. Her mouth and tongue attracted some fungus while hospitalized, so an infectious disease doctor prescribed antifungal meds and antibiotics to be included in Irene's TPN menu. Nevertheless …

Happy Interlude

During June 2010, after a two-year engagement, my son married the other Irene in his life. Tommy proposed to “his” Irene on bended knee at Disney’s Magic Kingdom, you may recall. Irene accepted “her” Tom’s proposal. I would fly north to witness my son get hitched.

Of course, my Irene could not make the trip. She was in the hospital. She was admitted the week before I left for the wedding. That was a wrenching decision: to leave or not to leave. My wife was in the hospital, and my son was getting married a thousand miles away. I made reservations before the doctors admitted Irene to the hospital. We did not realize she would be admitted at that time, but the hospital staff assured me—and Irene insisted—that everything was fine. The whole group, commanded by Irene, demanded that I keep my flight and hotel reservations and witness my son’s matrimony.

Thinking about it, Irene couldn’t have been in better hands. Her nurse attendants said she would probably be ready to be discharged when I returned, and there was nothing I could do at the moment anyway. After retrieving some toiletries and nightgowns and taking care of Dusty on a round trip to the house, I also brought back my camera to Irene’s bedside. I made a video of Irene in her hospital bed, sending a loving message to the happy couple.

Everyone up north was very disappointed she was unable to travel, including Irene, of course. But the happy couple came to Florida later, and we had a very nice celebration that included my Irene. By the way, my Irene loved it when I called her “my” Irene. And I loved it when she called me “her” Tom. Neither one of us was offended when the other used that possessive pronoun. We necessarily had to distinguish now that my son Tommy married an Irene. We all had the surname of Cooney.

Anyway, my Irene just started total parenteral nutrition a month or so earlier. While in the hospital, she received the TPN as prescribed, so there was no worry regarding her getting nutrition. She assured me that she could deliver the nutrition herself and could perform the flushing requirement if she was discharged before I returned. As I’ve indicated, it was not too difficult, but it is physically more difficult for the patient to get the right leverage for flushing. Important steps in the procedure had to be followed, that’s all. I worried a little. We’d been practicing for a month. I reviewed the procedure with her several times, and I felt confident she could do it, if necessary. As it happened, it wasn't necessary. I was away only four days. I had a suspicion the doctors would not discharge Irene until my return, but I still worried.

I arrived up north on Thursday evening. On Friday I collected my tuxedo that I was fitted for by phone. It wasn't too loose. I had my own shoes. We also attended the church for the rehearsal on Friday. The ceremony and reception were on Saturday.

Tommy and Irene beamed broad smiles from the beginning to the end of the ceremony at church and later at the reception, until Tommy smashed the first piece of wedding cake into Irene's face. She retaliated. Tradition is a stubborn thing to overcome. Promises to forgo such activities fall by the wayside when the couple is actually cutting the cake—and thinking bad thoughts. Those almost genetic thoughts force their way through the mind of at least one of the newly marrieds. In this case, it was Tommy's mind brewing the mischief. Everything was caught on camera, archived for future generations to view, chuckle, and comment upon.

"I couldn't resist. I just had to do it."

"My gown! My gown!"

Irene and her mother retreated to the ladies' room to make repairs. Who knows what was said between them at that time? Had Tommy damaged forever his relationship with his new mother-in-law? Not a chance, as it turned out.

Irene's parents are a great couple. If there was a moment of irritation at that time of the dress soiling, it was swiftly overcome by the general levity and happiness of the occasion. The families on both sides could not be more content with the choice of life's mate made by the bride and groom.

My brother filmed the entire ceremony at the church using my video camera. I was part of the wedding party and preoccupied. But being the archivist that I am, I captured the entire reception afterward and prepared copies for both families.

The next day, Sunday, when I landed in Orlando, I got a taxi from the airport. I called my Irene and told her I was on my way. I was anxious to get to the hospital to make sure everything was all right. I drove to the hospital and stayed overnight on a cot after taking care of Dusty. At the time, Irene's mother was staying with Tammy and the rest of the Holt household in Bradenton. I wanted to be with Irene. Irene was discharged on Monday, the next day. Timing was perfect.

06/21/2010: Tom is back. He stayed overnight. Discharged with orders for total parenteral nutrition along with antibiotics for tongue thrush to continue at home to include electrolytes, ertapenem, fluconazole 200 mg, mineral supplements, Protonix by mouth, 40 mg Carafate, zolpidem 12.5 mg at bedtime, docusate 150 mg/15 ml and weekly blood draws for labs by visiting RN. Tom administers it all through my port.—I. C.

When we got home, Irene and I watched the entire video of the ceremony and reception as we sat close to one another in our family room. Irene had tears in her eyes. She was so happy for the beautiful, newly wedded couple.

TPN Continued

Irene's sister, brother-in-law, and nephew—the Holt family—visited mid-summer 2010, and I went through the steps with Tammy of how to deliver TPN, just in case I got hit by a truck. I did it with my sister, too. I comforted them, noting their wide eyes, by saying I would be very careful crossing the street and driving and that a nurse would instruct them, if necessary.

When we returned from chemo sessions and I attached the TPN, lying in bed all those hours did not agree with Irene's style. Irene liked to be unattached as often as reasonable. She still needed the prescribed volume, though. To kill the time during those hours, I sat in a very comfortable lounge chair in our bedroom. I read to Irene, and when she would doze off, I'd read to myself.

I often retrieved my Bible that I studied during a theology class in night school in 1962, a couple years after I got out of the service: the Oxford Annotated Bible. (I can barely make out the price. It was either $5.95 or $15.95. What a bargain, either price!) It was edited by scholars and for the most part, they were neutral when referencing various treatises, comparisons, and archeological findings associated with biblical history. It was intended "to serve both a general reader and the student of the Bible." The margins were full of my own cryptic notes in my own handwriting. I barely understood them after almost fifty years. I couldn't deny the handwriting was mine, though.

I particularly enjoyed cross references with ancient historical and archeological facts. I think Irene liked it, too. One hears so many Bible quotes used popularly. It was always very interesting to see the quotes in total context with the ancient intended purposes. They were obviously different from its use in contemporary popular usage. The one in which we are cautioned to "Judge not lest ye be judged" comes to mind. To see for yourself, look it up in Matthew 7 and read the entire passage. Judgment of others is certainly not condemned as long as the one who judges is not being hypocritical.

And then of course there was my buddy Shakespeare. My recitations were probably the first time in Irene's life that someone read Shakespearean sonnets to her. Everyone should try it at least once.

At times, during those summer evenings, we would quietly look at each other. Our thoughts would intertwine, and we would read each other's minds. Lost in our own world, tears were always just below the surface and at the brink.

"Honey, remember when I carried you across the threshold of our motel room on I-95 on our way down here after our wedding?"

Irene nodded and her mouth opened slightly, but she couldn't quite utter an answer through her slightly trembling lips. She just reached for me to sit beside her on the bed. I left my chair. I went over and hugged her. We cried a little and held hands for a few minutes.

She finally smiled and teased me. "I thought you were going to drop me!"

We also watched a lot of the Cooking Channel, Irene's favorite. As time went by, I actually became more and more interested, especially in the challenges. *Restaurant Impossible* was riveting at times. And Irene, kind soul that she was, began to tolerate the History Channel, the Military Channel, Discovery Channel, and the Science Channel.

In the meantime, Irene had two more infusion sessions—conservative estimate: 148.

However, after a few months, the TPN was making her nauseated, an occasional side effect of TPN, along with all the other usual side effects from the ongoing chemo sessions. That created yet another problem. The chemo might be interfering with the healing of those stomach fistulas. Irene was feeling very bad. Then something else happened.

We were adjusting as much as possible to our situation, when Irene started to become quite jaundiced within a month of her last hospitalization. Her skin yellowed, her urine was very dark, and she experienced severe itching (puritis). Itching often accompanies jaundice.

I called the Direct Referral Center at Moffitt, and they told me to bring her to the hospital. They would have a bed waiting for her. After leaving a couple days of water and food for Dusty, we packed her toiletries and pajamas and went on our way. I also packed some overnight items in my little travel bag. This would be an extended stay, I was sure.

07/21/2010: Hospital admission through Moffitt Direct Referral Office with symptoms of jaundice, weakness, nausea, fever. Doctor surgically placed a biliary stent through my digestive tract. Amazing. I was knocked out for the procedure and was a little sore at first.—I. C.

Irene spent ten nights in the hospital this time. I slept over often and discovered a deli restaurant that served much better sandwiches than the hospital cafeteria. I returned home a couple times to take care of Dusty regularly. That was not a problem. I stayed overnight in our own bed and that replenished me to spend the next couple days on the hospital cot. That doesn't prepare anyone, however, for all the noise in a hospital during the wee hours of the night. It didn't matter. We were in the same room, at least.

After scans that determined Irene had a blockage in a biliary duct, she was taken downstairs to the endoscopy unit, where they anesthetized her and surgically removed the blocked area of the duct and replaced it with a stent; that is, an imitation piece of duct. The stent allowed proper draining through it. Surgeons decided to put in a long-lasting type stent, so Irene wouldn't have to undergo yet another procedure to replace the new stent anytime too soon. The medical staff didn't anticipate any trouble.

However, a year and a half later, she went through it again, except it wouldn't be quite as straightforward a procedure as this time.

While in the hospital, Irene developed pancreatitis and another fungal infection in her mouth and on her tongue. It took a few days extra of intravenous prescriptions in the hospital to control the problems. And due to that persistent mouth and tongue fungus, the prescription was changed to more powerful pharmaceuticals, along with another strong antibiotic.

07/31/2010: Discharged. Jaundice eventually cleared up by the time of discharge. TPN at home was to continue. Visiting nurse to collect and submit blood work each week, when she would change my port lead. Still problems eating. TPN including electrolytes, meropenem 2,000 mg over fifteen hours, micofungin 100 mg, along with regular TPN ingredients. Tom would add prescriptions to the TPN bag or line. Weekly labs by nurse also. I continue to experience some pain.—I. C.

The latest hospital stay was a long one. Between the hospital stay in early May (five days), last month's admission (eleven days), and this one (ten days), I slept on cots and traveled back and forth a lot of times. Irene, so far during this year of 2010, had a lot of admissions besides the last three. And there would be more.

At home, Irene continued to have a hard time forming words and eating for a while. I added those couple different antibiotics to Irene's main line through the Y junction to combat the infection after crushing them in a shot glass. The shot glass had a curved interior bottom so I could capture the full dose with the syringe after I liquefied it. None of the prescription was caught in a bottom crevice as when I first used the crusher container I'd bought for the purpose at the drugstore. The infection finally subsided.

At a scheduled appointment in the GI clinic in early August, the team continued the effort to fight the cancer by switching back to irinotecan and Erbitux. Irene became strong enough for chemo due to the benefit of external feeding.

That particular chemo combination was administered several years ago. The teams at both Fox Chase and at Moffitt used it. For a while, it was effective. Restarting a previously successful cocktail that has become less effective sometimes works well when tried again, after an earlier discontinuance.

Always busy, we traveled to Moffitt for three more chemo sessions (total: 151) and as usual, I hooked Irene up to TPN when we got home. She was exhausted, but that latest cocktail started having a beneficial effect in stopping the liver tumor from enlarging and spreading.

In our travels to and from the hospital, when Irene was up to it, we took advantage of a couple of little towns on our regular route. Sometimes we had a few hours before she had to be attached, especially if our chemo appointment was very early. We often left the house by 5:00 AM. We would be freed up in the late morning or early afternoon. We detoured through Plant City, the Strawberry Capital of the World, so they say, and I would fill up on strawberry shortcake. Irene would nibble.

Near Lake Alfred, there was a very cute teahouse. It served delicious pastries, including scones with Devonshire sauce. That was another stop we made on our way home. It provided one more chance to hold hands across the table.

TPN Discontinued

As the summer ended, Irene became more and more debilitated. She couldn't overcome a persistent, general malaise. She thought it was the antibiotics and the TPN. Irene told me she felt much better in the morning and as the day went on, before I attached her to TPN. But shortly after she was hooked to the TPN, at about 4:00 PM and during the night, she felt worse, particularly after I added the antibiotics and potassium.

The potassium created a burning sensation as soon as I administered it. I stopped it. The weekly lab reports reflected no ill effect due to my stopping the potassium. Evidently, she didn't need that supplement any longer—at that time. She would need it again in a little while, along with more magnesium.

During this period, Irene took up to ten Imodium a day for relief of diarrhea. She'd lost more than twelve pounds since her last weigh-in. She was eating a little soft food throughout the day, such as creamed spinach, mashed potatoes, and baby food that I picked up at the supermarket. She tried to eat other foods, too. She wanted to get off the TPN.

She thought she might try pizza and celery with cream cheese. They made her vomit. Irene kept getting nauseated. She threw up after eating roughage such as salads and fruit too. So she just ate the soft foods. She wanted to be rid of the whole TPN apparatus. It was making her very sick. She also became very anemic again.

During a chemo visit in late August, the doctors noticed Irene was becoming very weak with all that vomiting and diarrhea. They told us to temporarily stop the TPN after we finished the three bags we had left. They notified the supplier to hold off the next shipment. They told us to give it a try—to see if Irene could eat enough by mouth to gain a little weight and begin to feel better. At that time, the doctors would decide whether or not Irene needed to remain on continuous TPN or if she could eat enough calories during the day so she could stay off it.

At our next regular visit in early September 2010, with a big, disarming smile, Irene again requested the team to take her completely off TPN. I hadn't hooked her up to the TPN for a couple weeks by this time. It had been temporarily stopped in late August 2010, due to Irene's continual vomiting and diarrhea. She said she would try to eat more soft food to get enough nutrition. She wanted to also stop taking all those antibiotics for treating those ugly fistulas in her stomach. She felt the prescriptions were making her sick too. She hoped and prayed. We both did. She wanted to gain some weight.

At the following infusion appointment, September 14, 2010, prior to going upstairs for chemo, the team relented when confronted with Irene's convincing smile—she could stop the TPN, but not until they sat her in a lounge chair and delivered a unit of potassium and a unit of magnesium over the next couple hours. They wanted her to be ready to better handle the infusion scheduled for that day. When Irene was finished with her chemo for the day, we firmed up the next chemo date in a couple weeks: September 28, 2010.

In the meantime, however, she became dehydrated again, due to the vomiting and severe diarrhea. We phoned. She was instructed to come to the Direct Referral Center. We drove to Moffitt, where a hospital bed was prepared for her.

09/23/2010: Admitted to Moffitt hospital again. They kept me overnight just to be rehydrated. I was told to follow up with my primary oncologist before getting chemo, as scheduled on 09/28/2010.—I. C.

Enteral Feeding Tube

When we returned on September 28, 2010, chemo was canceled for that day. Irene was too weak. After a long discussion and with Irene's approval, the medical team decided to use a surgically inserted feeding tube instead of TPN for nutrition. They wanted chemo to be able to start up again, after the procedure.

The operation required a very complex, major surgical procedure in Irene's case. The previous surgery in the area around her stomach and the two fistulas complicated things. The holes had healed somewhat but were still unresolved. The entrance site for the tube would have to be in the small intestine (jejunum) instead of the normal insertion in the stomach cavity, because of the fistulas in Irene's stomach.

Compared to describing the process of TPN and its dispensing, I discovered that trying to write the following description of the enteral feeding tube, its insertion and subsequent delivery of nutrition into Irene's system was something like a how-to for tying my shoelaces—very intricate.

Imagine a small incision less than a half inch long that the surgeon created in Irene's abdomen on her left side while she was under anesthesia. A clear hollow tube, also less than a half inch in diameter, came out of that incision, dangling about seven or eight inches onto her belly. There also was another twelve inches or so of tubing inside her, worming down through her small intestine (or jejunem).

Average length of the small intestine is twenty-two or twenty-three feet long, but females actually have a small intestine about nine to twelve inches *longer* than males. It is, on average, about an inch in diameter.

The beginning of the small intestine, as it leaves the stomach, is the duodenum. The duodenum begins at the stomach exit. The next section of your small intestine, following the duodenum, is the jejunem. The rest of it—all the way until it gets to the colon—is the ileum.

The ileum is the longest part of the small intestine. The cecum connects the ileum to the colon, which itself is nearly five feet long. That's where the process of waste elimination begins. The colon's several parts end at the rectum. Irene had about eighteen inches of the transverse, descending, and sigmoid sections of her colon removed in her very first cancer operation.

Basically, the esophagus, the stomach, the small intestine, and the colon make up the digestive system. The stomach and small intestine is where most of the food gets broken down and absorbed to provide nutrition.

Because of the unhealed fistulas, combined with a slight kink in her intestine in the area near the exit of Irene's stomach due to a previous surgery in that area, Irene had a very difficult time ingesting food of any kind in the beginning, after that radio-embolization. She then went necessarily onto the TPN. Gradually, she was only able to slightly improve her intake because of pain and vomiting. The TPN eventually caused too much nausea. It was discontinued. But the medical team wanted to get Irene healthy enough so she could continue the chemo infusions. The team felt an urgency to continue the chemo. Irene needed external nutrition, at least temporarily; hopefully, not permanently.

I think most feeding tubes are probably inserted into a patient's stomach, usually because there is an eating problem with the esophagus, throat, or mouth, or other inability to eat. The term used for such a tube is G-tube, the G standing for gastro or stomach. The stomach is a relatively large cavity. There's usually no trouble dispensing nutrition directly into someone's stomach and allowing normal digestion from that point downstream. The incision site may weep or leak, which can be troublesome, but it is usually infrequent. It is different with the J-tube, one that is inserted into the small intestine, the jejunem.

Irene was admitted to the hospital on September 28. All the many preparatory screenings were completed by October 6, eight days later. She was wheeled into the surgical suite, where she stayed for several hours. The J-tube was inserted into her jejunem, which is only about an inch in diameter—not nearly as large as a stomach cavity.

09/28/2010: Hospital admission to Moffitt Cancer Center through Direct Referral Office for insertion of J-tube.—I. C.

10/06/2010: After scans and prepping all done, tube will be surgically inserted into my small intestine. At the same time the doctors will create a pathway (G-J tube) from the bottom of my stomach directly to the jejunem, upstream of the J-tube, so that I might be able to sometimes experience the pleasure of eating.—I. C.

Observe from Irene's notation above, the surgeons (two of them) made an incision in the very bottom of Irene's stomach and another in her jejunem immediately adjacent to her duodenum. Why? Because the doctors did not want Irene to become totally dependent on the external feeding. They linked Irene's stomach directly to her jejunem upstream from the other half-inch site that accommodated the entry for the feeding tube itself. If she were able to ingest anything without getting sick, the food would empty into her small intestine from that low point in her stomach, avoiding the troubled area at the exit of her stomach. That short connector was a G-J tube, a pathway from Irene's stomach to her jejunem. The G-J tube was very short, but to place it, they had to open Irene up and fully expose her intestines, because they had to manipulate them. It was a procedure within a procedure.

The surgeons encouraged Irene to eat as tolerated. They even prescribed an appetite enhancer. Initially, it all looked promising for Irene.

The main tube, through which the external nutrition would flow, was placed several inches downstream from the exit of her stomach, duodenum, and the G-J tube. The feeding tube itself, the J-tube, snaked for another foot farther down into Irene's small intestine. The tube was flexible and could conform through the contours and turns of her small intestine as necessary. At the open end of the tube, out of which the nutrition flowed into her system, less than an inch from that opening, there was a small balloon. The balloon could be inflated and deflated with a tiny amount of saline solution through a Y connector, using a syringe. Its purpose was to prevent the tube from escaping the incision site. It was designed to catch the end of the tube, preventing it from falling out of her abdomen, especially during sleep or unconsciousness.

You can see how that additional space taken up by the balloon, when inflated inside the jejunem, might further restrict the flow of any food and digestive juices around and through the narrow one-inch channel of Irene's small intestine. That blockage and restriction caused severe leakage from her jejunem up onto Irene's abdomen through that small half-inch incision that accommodated the tube entering Irene's abdomen. Food and digestive juices continuously escaped the incision site and caused Irene to suffer very irritating, red, and raw soreness around the entry site. It gave her discomfort for months and months.

Eventually, after a phone consultation with one of the surgeons, I made several attempts at the optimal inflation of the balloon, trying to observe whether there was greater or lesser leakage around the small incision site. Finally, the surgeon told me to deflate the balloon completely to allow the freest flow through the narrow channel in Irene's small intestine. The surgeon told me to make sure I secured the tube to Irene's abdomen with well-anchored bandaging.

That half-inch incision through which the J-tube was inserted into Irene's jejunem caused a big problem. The fit of the tube in the hole was not tight enough, so the leakage was constant. A purse stitch tightened the area surrounding the tube but only briefly. Too many purse stitches, and the tissue around the opening deteriorated due to too many needle punctures. The skin might tear between each suture. That leakage allowed the escaping fluids to soil her clothes and bed sheets.

I want to make a distinction between the large surgical incision that allowed access to Irene's intestines to insert the G-J tube and the small, leaky one that the external tube needed to make entry into Irene's small intestine. The larger surgical cut on Irene's abdomen that opened up her abdomen so the doctors could gain access to manipulate her intestines was going to take a longer time to heal.

10/11/2010 and 10/12/2010: While in the hospital, Psychosocial & Palliative Medicine Program consulted. Fentanyl patch, 75 mcg/hr;

and lidoderm with one patch on twelve hours and then off twelve hours. Continue Dilaudid.—I. C.

I went home every other day to take care of Dusty and tend to the pool. I never really minded the drive to Moffitt. I could daydream while I was driving. I enjoyed seeing the sun's reflection in the form of a cross on that dome midway between our home and the hospital.

10/13/2010: Discharged with my new tube hanging out of my stomach. Nutrition is Jevity 1.2, five 8-ounce cans a day, with frequent flushes. They team taught us the process. Tom can handle it. I'm able to nibble a little bit.—I. C.

Irene wouldn't be released for another week after the surgery, a total of fifteen days from admission to discharge. We followed up with the surgeon later in the month. There was a lot of leakage from the small J-tube incision site from the start, especially if Irene managed to swallow anything solid. She once tried to eat some licorice swirls that she craved. Her skin, all around the tube's incision, turned black. I cleaned it up. Irene had the same mess with brownies, just a different color.

It required constant replenishing of new, very large absorbent bandages each time. I went to the local medical supply store and stocked up with various sizes of bandages and ointments to take care of the leakage and soreness around the tube insertion area. The tube sight was getting very raw. I made a slit from the edge of the bandage so I could slide it around the tube; then I cut a small circular hole to the size of the circumference of the tube so it would fit snugly.

10/29/2010: Friday. Local hospital ER. I was having heavy leakage from my feeding tube, as usual. Tom called Moffitt, and they told him to take me to the ER for a purse stitch and call them if any problem arose. The PA on duty did not know how to do a purse stitch. Tom got her in touch with Moffitt, and the PA talked on the phone with Moffitt. The PA did a single stitch and told me to follow up at Moffitt.—I. C.

11/01/2010: Monday. Another trip to Moffitt. The repair was made with several purse stitches by the surgeon.—I. C.

11/09/2010: Still leaking. At my next appointment, Moffitt nurse placed an ostomy bag over it and scheduled inserting a larger-diameter tube to try to limit leakage from the site. Nurse showed Tom how to cut the adherent side of the ostomy bags to accommodate the tube when he has to replace them every day, sometimes more often. Expensive at the medical supply store. Too much trouble to submit to insurance company right now.—I. C.

While all this leaking and discomfort was happening, other problems arose regularly. I delivered the nutrition over fifteen hours, as prescribed. I flushed periodically with huge syringes that I filled from bottles of saline. I wanted to prevent clogging. I did it every time I added a medication too.

Administering the nutrition required weaving the main line through a pump. Most of the time, the pump did the job—in the beginning. When Irene moved around during the night, the main line crimped causing the pump to set off a loud, repeating beep. It sounded off regularly. It's that same beep you hear in the hospital to alert the nurse that the flow has stopped or the meds have emptied, signaling it's time to replenish. The shrill beep during the night annoyed us, to say the least, and intruded immensely on our sleep.

That's not all! Sometimes I couldn't find out why it was beeping. I'd flush and flush again in case it was a clogging problem that the pump was sensing. I was on the phone with the supplier, entering secret proprietary codes into the pump to increase the flow rate or reduce the chance of clogging yet maintain a sufficient rate to deliver enough nutrition to Irene.

It was challenging to deal with the leaks, ensure the site stayed clean, give Irene her meds and injections at the right time, fill the supply bag, make sure the cases of Jevity liquid nutrition were available, and take care of several other necessities and chores, but we handled it.

Finally, I was able to diagnose the problem with the beeping and clogging. The darned pump was malfunctioning. I arranged for a new pump, and the process went much smoother from that point. It was very frustrating for a couple of weeks. We tried to stay optimistic, but it required focus. We didn't need any unnecessary distractions. We kept busy going to the local ER and to Moffitt, mostly due to the feeding tube and its related leakage problems.

11/22/2010: Tube still leaking. They decided to finally replace it. The tube was replaced in Moffitt, radiology, with a larger diameter.—I. C.

We weren't done yet. The human body has some strange methods to overcome restrictions in the digestive track. The tidbits of food Irene was able to take by mouth were finding the pathway created by that small shortcut tube (G-J) that the doctors had placed, connecting the bottom of her stomach directly to her small intestine. That was a good thing. It was several inches upstream from the main J-tube.

Once the food exited that route, however, it was being stopped up at the location where the J-tube entered her jejunem, farther downstream in her small intestine. Well, the digestive juices also ate their way up through Irene's abdominal wall into her belly. In addition to the primary leak, the acids erupted onto her skin a half inch from the actual insertion site in the northwest quadrant. It actually looked like a very large boil at first, and then it broke. Irene was incredibly frustrated. Everyone was flustered, even the doctors.

Irene's main J-tube occupied about a third of the inch-diameter space inside her jejunem—a tube within a tube. That J-tube, inside, went another twelve inches along the inside of her small intestine—the space for food to travel was restrictive. If there was a logjam, there was no place for the debris to go but up, through the very tissue of Irene's abdominal wall. It had to get around the rest of the J-tube that was inside Irene's jejunem, but it couldn't. It has only two-thirds of the normal space. It backed up. And that small balloon that was normally used to anchor the tube within the abdomen caused additional blockage until I deflated it completely. There were now two leaking openings on poor Irene's abdomen. One created itself—not a surgeon's scalpel. Just imagine!

11/26/2010: Tom took me to local ER again. New tube didn't help. Still leaking. Same as before. There is leakage of greenish material surrounding my J-tube and another eruption that is leaking brownish fluid. Mepilex Border 18 cm x 18 cm applied by a PA. Held several hours. Thanksgiving yesterday. Couldn't eat much.—I. C.

11/27/2010: Saturday. Released from local hospital after several tests. I had a fever. As usual, told to follow up with Moffitt Cancer Center, GI clinic.—I. C.

12/01/2010: Wednesday. They replaced the tube again in Moffitt, radiology. There's still too much play within the tube hole. The other leak in my stomach is still oozing, too. Tom cleans it up and puts balm and Desitin to try to make it feel better. Uses ostomy bags he bought from supply store in St. Cloud. I can't do it myself because I can't see it from the right angle. Tom can see it directly. Nothing helps. It burns terribly and soils the bedclothes and my nightgowns.—I. C.

The surgeon at Moffitt instructed me on how to probe, clean out, and then pack the channel of that "volcano." I had to do it daily. I'd take a Q-tip and clean it and then take a strip of quarter-inch ribbon sterile gauze about three inches long, roll it up, and then push it into that nasty volcano's opening to a depth of a third of an inch. Then I'd cover the wound with a patch. I used paper tape. It saved Irene some pain and agony as she contended with the frequent probing, patching, and re-taping.

Inspiring everyone who knew of her predicament, Irene handled all her pain and disappointment right in stride. She still smiled and retained her sense of humor through it all. Take, for example, the little balloon, located at the end of the tube where the nutrition entered into Irene's intestine, which was completely deflated per the surgeon's orders. One night, about a week into December, I heard Irene yelling from the bathroom,

"Tom! Tom! The tube came out!"

I scrambled into the master bath's commode room, where Irene looked panicked, holding the tube in her lap with a frightened look on her pretty face (picture a frown with a smile). I turned the pump off and quickly donned rubber gloves. I told her,

"Okay, honey. Don't worry. Let me have it. Wheel the pole back to bed and lie down. I'll put it back in. Remember, they told me if it came out and I got it right away, I could weave it back inside you."

If it was out for a long time—for example, if she woke up and found it beside her, and we didn't know when it had come out—we'd have to go to the ER and have it put back, because the incision site might have closed.

Irene calmed down right away and reclined on our bed, waiting for me to perform. Then she smiled with a twinkle in her eye, saying,

"Okay, Dr. Cooney. Have your way with me."

"Honey, you've always trusted me completely. I love you for that."

She continued smiling and then blew a bawdy kiss up at me.

I carefully placed the business end of the long, flexible tube back into the incision site and started gently and slowly weaving it through Irene's small intestine. Nice and easy did it. I could feel the curvature of her jejunem as the head of the tube snaked its way farther and farther inside her body downstream. I stopped when there was about seven inches still outside her belly. I anchored it the best I could with tape to lock the tube in place.

I hooked her up to the feeding apparatus again and asked, "How did that feel, honey?"

"Wow! Wonderful! Just wonderful! If I were a smoker, I'd light up a cigarette."

After a spontaneous laugh, I smiled and said,

"You're funny, honey."

It's very difficult to keep Irene's sense of humor suppressed for long.

12/13/2010: Feeding tube has been very problematic. They replaced it again—third time! Plus, my regular doses of biweekly chemo sessions continued the last several weeks. Because of years of chemo, the regularly prescribed doses leave me very sick most of the time. Reduced dosage levels are currently recommended. Another diagnostics study. I believe it was for mapping that extra "volcanic" eruption (fistula path). They might make a plug to stop the leaking. They may give Tom Super Glue to stop the leakage.—I. C.

12/15/2010: A scan showed slight increase in the size of the nodule in my liver. The oncologist, in conference with the surgeon, wanted to offer me options using FOLFOX instead of the current cocktail—irinotecan and Erbitux. My doctor preferred FOLFOX because it had helped me quite a bit in the past. But oxaliplatin causes me problems. They may decide to infuse FOLFOX at a slower rate (over twelve hours) and reduce the dosage also. We'll see about it next year. I have an appointment right after New Year's with the surgeon to check out the tube site and then the oncologist on January 11.—I. C.

Irene did have two more chemo sessions during the preceding time frame. Fortunately, her liver tumors responded to the chemo. That was good news on the cancer front, even though the discomfort surrounding the enteral feeding tube was still very problematic.

The doctors didn't want too much delay in delivering the irinotecan and Erbitux. They continued chemo through December. That brought the total to 156 by the end of the year. We still had a battle going on, so no one wanted to just stand by, including Irene. She wanted that cocktail. She started to gain some weight too.

They checked the liver nodules and the healing of the fistulas with regular scans. Doctors also ordered a fistulagram to map the shape and path of that other very unusual eruption on Irene's abdomen. They considered ordering a custom-made plug to stop it from leaking so much. We measured the amount of discharge regularly in an ostomy bag that I secured over the site and noticed that it was finally decreasing.

Very gradually, even the fistulas began to heal, including the two on the inside of her stomach caused by the radio-embolization and the weird one that erupted near the J-tube incision site. But the J-tube site incision was still leaking most of the time. We dealt with it. They kept increasing the size of the tube until ultimately, it was the largest size available.

Another time or two, Irene and I engaged in the little saucy banter when I had to reinsert the tube. It was lighthearted fun.

The team members wanted to fight the cancer, but they were concerned the chemo was retarding the healing of the tube's insertion site and the fistulas. They considered using oxaliplatin again but in a different manner. The process of lowering the dose, during a twelve-hour rate of flow, is termed *desensitization*. That was at least a fifteen-hour day. But we'd had very long days before. However, we both thought that particular cocktail could come later. For now, we wanted to see what happened with the next scans. We'd go from there. It was time to give Irene a well-deserved treatment break. What was happening to her was exasperating, as you can imagine.

Doctors continued to monitor the leakage and changed the tube to an ever larger diameter, when necessary. The largest tube available didn't solve the problem. When it became my job to change the tube, they supplied me with slightly firmer red tubes that didn't kink as often, causing that annoying beep. It also saved us the frequent trips to exchange the tube. The surgeon had confidence I could do it.

However, there was a little trick to using an X-ACTO blade to incise the standard opening at the end of the red tube. I could increase the flow rate a bit and decrease the chance of clogging. I had regularly used X-ACTO blades during my train and airplane modeling days. The surgeon showed me how to do it without ruining the tube. I had no problem.

As each day passed in December, Irene was eating a little bit more. We still had hope. The ever expanding team members considered clinical trials at that time. The tube site needed constant cleansing and new dressings. And I still had to position the ostomy bags around the tube by cutting a slit and a small-diameter hole to accommodate the tube. All those supplies entailed a lot of out-of-pocket expense. I thanked my lucky stars I could afford to pay.

12/22/2010: Our last visit of the year. Tom asked if surgery to cut out the disease in my liver is an option. We were told that surgery is no longer an option in my case. I've gotten to the point that I would jump at surgery, but I can't have it anymore. We'll just have to hope the chemo works. I set up my next appointment for 01/11/2011.—I. C.

The surgeon told us to contact her in a week or two if the skin around the eruption did not completely heal. She could offer us some tissue glue (actually, Super Glue) in an attempt to solidify the fistula closure. Irene was going to resume chemo after the holidays and the glue might help to avoid leakage when Irene restarted her chemotherapy the next month. The fistula plug was the best option to stop the oozing, but that might take a few weeks to get, as it had to be ordered. It would be custom-made at an outside facility.

At our last visit of the year, the surgeon reviewed the scans with Irene and me and confirmed that there were no new lesions and only minimal to moderate increase in the liver metastasis. The infusions were paying off. A few weeks' interlude from chemotherapy should not have a significant impact on the progression of Irene's disease. We desperately needed the break.

For the rest of the year, Irene still had signs of that persistent fungal infection on her tongue. I still added the prescribed meds to the feeding container, along with potassium again. This time, I put the potassium in with the fluid nutrition bag so, by the time it got to Irene's system, it was diluted without losing effectiveness.

Christmas came. Despite Irene's diarrhea, overall malaise, and other side effects from the chemo and the feeding tube, we were still able to drive to Bradenton to see Irene's mother and the rest of her family. The reflection of the cross on that dome-shaped building followed us as we passed, going to and coming from Bradenton. What did it mean?

We couldn't stay long, but I could always delay hooking Irene to the feeding tube for several hours until we returned home. It was no worse than being late for supper. Irene was beginning to gain a little weight by this time. We possibly could skip a day occasionally, as long as Irene continued to gain some weight. At that time, however, we stuck to the program.

As usual, gifts were exchanged and a great meal was shared by all in attendance. Irene was able to sample everything without any major distress. That was a very good sign.

Irene's mother was in a good, merry mood, kibitzing with her grandson, Irene's nephew. It uplifted Maria into the holiday spirit. Irene felt cheerful too.

"Merry Christmas, Tom."

"And the same to you, my dear."

"You look like you're putting on a little weight, honey."

"Yes! Isn't that great?"

I love her in that sky blue outfit, I thought. *It brings out the blossom on her cheeks. Her strength is amazing. Everyone loves hearing her laugh and enjoying herself.*

As we were leaving and I gazed at Irene enjoying herself, I reached for her hand and as usual, she clasped mine. As she inched toward me, I took her close and softly placed my right hand to that blossomed cheek.

She bent her head slightly toward my hand and caressed my hand with her own.

“I love you, honey,” I said softly.

“Hold me close, dear.”

“That’s very easy for me to do. I love holding you, Irene.”

Irene said her rosary on the way home from her sister’s. She seemed at peace. I kept quiet. I loved this woman so much. It was a little too dark to see our cross on the domed building by the time we drove home.

“Next time,” I told her. “Don’t worry, honey. We’re on I-4 a lot. We’ll see it next time.”

Chapter Nine

The Continuing Leakage Problem

The holidays came and went. The tube incision site was still leaking. The bed sheets and Irene's nightgowns and street clothes were all stained with bilious fluids. Irene was scheduled to resume chemotherapy on January 11, 2011, but by the first weekend in January, we noticed that a circle of infection had appeared around the small J-tube incision site. The ring was more than an inch in diameter. In addition, Irene had a slight fever. I called Moffitt and arranged for a visit on Tuesday, January 4, with the surgeon who'd inserted the J-tube.

01/04/2011: Right after New Year's, the incision site looked infected. Tom called the surgeon who told us to come in.—I. C.

That red ring filled in over a short period. Irene said it itched and was very tender to the touch. Even so, there was some progress to report. She was gaining weight. Irene was also tolerating a daily oral intake of certain foods, supplemented with the J-tube feedings. She still had the general nausea and diarrhea, so her J-tube feed prescriptions were changed again to increase the fiber content of the Jevity. Irene also told the doctor about the burning around the J-tube site after I administered the potassium elixir through the J-tube's catheter. All things considered, she was ready and even eager to start chemo again.

01/12/2011: I had a full strength chemo session. It gave me severe side effects, diarrhea especially. Can't eat much by mouth right now either. Nevertheless, I scheduled another session for two weeks from now. I want to get this stuff out of my body as fast as I can.—I. C.

Irene was infused for the 157th time. It again gave her pretty bad side effects. It didn't stop her, though.

01/26/2011: I had another full-strength chemo session. New eruption of the cutaneous fistula near the tube insertion site after this session (probably caused by chemo strength).—I. C.

Two weeks later, Irene had her 158th full-strength chemo infusion, and it again gave her pretty bad side effects. The sensitivity to cold in her hands, fingers, feet, and toes was causing Irene a lot of pain. The nausea and vomiting continued without any relief. Irene dealt with mouth sores regularly too. The fistula that erupted near the tube insertion site was still oozing fluid. It was depressing for Irene to continually experience the leakage from both locations. It was not a very jubilant fifty-eighth birthday for Irene toward the end of January. But friends and relatives knew little of Irene's discomfort. She was quiet about it, except between the two of us.

As an aside: I recently had a bout of what I believe was food poisoning. I experienced violent vomiting and diarrhea for two days. And for the following day or two, I was very cautious. I stayed in bed. I felt miserable. While lying in bed, I reminded myself that I was sick for just a few days. Irene had felt this way for years and years, with only relatively brief periods free of nausea, vomiting, diarrhea, and many other symptoms. My momentary illness reinforced my respect for Irene's fortitude and her ability to smile and suffer in silence. She was an amazing human being. When you think you are having a bad day, think about Irene's bad days.

In early February, I rushed Irene to the local ER. She was admitted into the hospital again.

02/04/2011 to 02/06/2011: Admitted to local hospital after Tom took me to the ER. Overall weakness and dehydration. Also, severe tube leakage and difficulty breathing. I was kept Saturday for observation and low potassium level. My feeding tube was not used or irrigated. Finally, a GI doctor attempted to unclog my tube because the floor nurses failed to do so while I was in the hospital. He couldn't clear it. He recommended I have it replaced at Moffitt. Also, Tom and his sister, who were visiting me in the hospital, both thought my right leg was slightly swollen. I was released Sunday, 02/06/2011, when, after X-rays of chest, they did not find anything else and recommended follow-up at Moffitt Cancer Center. I was glad to get out of that hospital.—I. C.

We had a regularly scheduled appointment three days after Irene was released from the local hospital. We simply waited.

02/09/2011: At my next regular appointment at Moffitt, the following Wednesday, physician assistant, GI clinic, ordered a Doppler of my right leg after feeling a little swelling. The Doppler discovered a clot that the local hospital missed. Fragmin (10,000 units) was prescribed and has since eliminated swelling. Reduction in units was mentioned and/or less expensive thinner.—I. C.

02/09/2011: Also, same day, PA recommended and arranged (she is good and on top of things) to upsize feeding tube to a #22 as it was leaking badly. Replacement is a very short procedure with no anesthesia needed. If the tube comes out at home (and it did), as long as it is right away, Tom just puts it back in. If a larger size is needed, the doctor would order and insert it.—I. C.

As I mentioned before, the surgeon finally decided that fully deflating the anchor balloon at the forward end of the J-tube; restricting oral intake, and nourishing only with J-tube Jevity feedings, would result in healing of the fistula that caused all the leakage. She was right. The nuisance volcano stopped erupting and was starting to slowly resolve after we followed the surgeon's advice. Irene was also gradually able to eat more and more solid foods to supplement the tube feedings.

The tube incision site still leaked, however, just as much as always, in spite of some healing around the site. I continued to use absorbent bandages and the ostomy bags. But based on the latest scans that showed Irene's disease was worsening, the surgeon saw no reason why Irene shouldn't resume chemotherapy as soon as possible.

03/07/2011: Latest CAT scan. Liver tumor has enlarged and also spread into head of pancreas and lymph nodes.—I. C.

03/16/2011: Chemo was restarted and completed at regular strength (severe side effects). Discussion with doctors about the "quality vs. quantity" decision that people in my situation must make at some point. Palliative and supportive hospice care was also discussed. Doctors say that chemo is still available but reduced dosage is recommended to alleviate severe side effects. We were told again that there would be no more surgery in the future. I opted to continue chemo infusions. Tom and I want "quantity."—I. C.

During the visit in mid-March, we discussed the possibility of removing the feeding tube completely and stopping chemo. The tube interfered so much with her quality of life, and she was disgusted with it. It contributed to Irene's developing an overall depression. Tears were close behind any sad event that she witnessed, even if she was not intimately associated with it. We tried to stay away from tragic news on television.

The depression revealed itself in subtle ways. As an example of Irene's ability to feel deeply and her pervasive melancholy, you might remember my mentioning that a Ukrainian woman, who had a home in another subdivision within the same golfing community, was visiting from Michigan. She and her husband were friends of ours. The woman stopped at our home to say hello.

Her husband did not accompany her on this particular trip, which was unusual. When Irene asked about his absence, the woman said that he was having health problems and at the last minute said he wasn't feeling up to the trip, even though it was going to be a short one. She added that he had a protrusion in his abdomen. Irene was aware that this friend had lost her first husband to cancer.

Immediately, Irene's eyes filled with tears and, saying nothing, reached over and hugged the distraught woman. Each woman felt sympathy for the other. The three of us were from a smaller world than most. We each understood how tears could easily flow. It wasn't difficult for each of the three of us to cry, considering what was going on in our lives.

During that quality versus quantity discussion with the medical team in mid-March 2011, the team repeated that Irene would not be getting any more surgery in the future. That meeting seemed to be a turning point, at least in our minds. But true to form, Irene bravely wanted to continue chemo. She refused to give up.

Irene had a unit of intravenous magnesium during that visit, and she also just had her 159th infusion. On one hand, the oncologist was afraid the tube incision might not heal if the tube was taken out. On the other hand, the surgeon was concerned that once removed, Irene would have to depend completely on oral eating—there could not be another tube placement. The surgeon added, however, that she thought no problem would develop with healing, even if Irene resumed infusions.

The surgeon strongly suggested that Irene restart chemo at reduced-strength dosages and continue the fight against the disease. The surgeon agreed to approve removing the tube whenever Irene was ready. Irene decided to take some time to think about her situation. It was a huge decision. It was almost a "to be or not to be" decision, if you think about it. I could see the years of roller-coaster ups and downs had taken a huge toll on Irene. No one else saw it, though.

03/29/2011: Chemo session at reduced strength (mild side effects). I got a unit of magnesium, too, before chemo. The small volcano fistula remains closed. It seems that it is not much affected by the lower doses of chemo. I am able to eat a small meal or two a day to supplement the tube feeding.—I. C.

Irene ended March 2011, with her 160th chemo session. She was insistent on continuing infusions, albeit at reduced potency. Her side effects were manageable with her regularly prescribed various medications, which were to be taken at different times of the day. Taking those meds never stopped, not even when she was unable to take them orally. I would crush them into a powder, liquefy them, and administer them directly through the main feed lines or inject them into the 2,000 ml bag containing the nutrition. Either way, she benefitted from them.

Here's a partial list of Irene's medications on March 29, 2011. Realize, though, that as her disease worsened, medications varied. Generics were used in most cases:

Compazine 10 mg every six hours for nausea
Carafate 1 gram orally every six to eight hours
Hydromorphone (Dilaudid) 4 mg every two hours for pain
Lorazepam (Ativan) .5 mg every six hours for anxiety, as needed
Lomotil (atropine-diphenoxylate) every four hours, as needed
Zolpidem (Ambien) 12.5 mg at bedtime
Ondansetron (Zofron) 4 mg every four hours, as needed
Lidoderm patch daily to abdomen: twelve hours on, twelve hours off
Fentanyl 75 mcg/hr: every seventy-two hours, as needed (later, 100 mcg/hr.)
Metoclopramide (Reglan) 10 mg three times a day, as needed
Jevity 1.2: five 8-ounce cans a day, via J-tube
Fragmin: 10,000 units 3 ml daily; PA will change to either a lower dose or generics (warfarin or enoxaparin)

Tylenol Arthritis, as needed
Prevacid SoluTab 30 mg once daily

From this point forward, additional medications were administered through Irene's port, both prior to and after infusions, intending to alleviate the chemo's associated side effects. They helped a little but not that much. Irene still had severe nausea, vomiting, diarrhea, mouth sores, the painful itching in her hands and feet and several other usual side effects. Fatigue was one of her major concerns. She felt herself tiring and spending more time in bed each day. It was always on her mind.

To summarize briefly: after a full year, though improved, the internal stomach fistulas had not completely healed. In addition, Irene's last CAT scan in early March 2011, showed encroachment of a liver tumor into the head of her pancreas and the involvement of several lymph nodes in her abdominal area. Imagine getting that news when she was already feeling low.

In addition, four other reduced-strength chemo sessions were tentatively scheduled for April 11, April 26, May 10, and May 24, 2011. That included numbers 161, 162, 163, and 164, when completed. CAT scans follow intermittently, usually monthly, to determine the value of continuing the treatment. At this point, within a month or so, Irene would decide whether or not to discontinue the chemo and/or remove the feeding tube.

Additional Worries: Insurance Search

Before I continue describing Irene's treatment, which picked up in April 2011, I want to mention our particular medical insurance situation. Everyone who fights cancer has to continually think about money.

I gave critical thought to where in this book I should mention finances and medical costs. Rather than sprinkling comments here and there, I believe it is best to devote these paragraphs, arranged compactly, to describe the subject. It will provide perspective regarding the additional anxiety a family deals with while a loved one is a cancer patient.

At this time, we were also dealing with Irene's continuing problematic treatments and leakage around her J-tube incision site. Remember, Irene's five year insurance coverage after retirement from the police department was going to expire June 1, 2011. By the end of March 2011, I started a desperate search to replace her coverage. Her pre-existing condition would be a hurdle to overcome. We had to face the question of coverage only during this particular period of Irene's care and life.

There were no concerns about my coverage. I was over sixty-five and eligible for Medicare. I only needed to enhance my coverage with a Medicare supplemental plan that offered prescription co-pays. My medical insurance plan (Plan F) was the best offered, and I could afford it. There were no worries about my coverage.

While we continued looking for insurance, Irene's chemo sessions eventually resumed.

04/11/2011: Irinotecan and Erbitux again and of course, my usual unit of magnesium before chemo. My insurance plan requires us to move back to the five-county Philadelphia area to get coverage from Law Enforcement Health Benefits. Tom checking it out. It's a worry.—I. C.

The decision to move became moot, though we didn't know it at the time. (Today, under the same plan, a retiree is not required to move back to Pennsylvania. Rules change!)

I personally went to several insurance offices, including those representing big and small providers. I was told by many representatives of companies that they didn't have anything available. I made numerous phone calls.

All the while, Irene was worrying. The last thing in the world Irene wanted was to be responsible for causing huge outlays of money and assets. She shed tears over the problem that she thought she was creating. That's the way she was. She never placed herself first; it was always others. That's why I married her, after all. She was completely unselfish.

We were far from being penniless, thank God. I had done nicely with investments and the business.

How could we preserve both a legacy to my children and attend to possibly millions more dollars in medical expenses? Irene loved my sons. Sadly, she had no biological children of her own. She didn't want my sons to lose what I had worked a lifetime for and had nest-egged for them.

In the spring of 2011, I told my sons what we were considering and our plight. They told me to take care of Irene, whatever it took. They said I should worry only about Irene and get her the very best care. They loved Irene. They had known and loved her for ten years by this time. They would manage their own futures (and they have, very nicely). I was proud of them for saying that. It lightened my burden.

Irene wanted to know if she was eligible for any kind of aid. We spoke to a social worker at Moffitt Cancer Center. Irene would choke up. Lately, she would cry and weep easily. I always tried to comfort her. No amount of my cajoling or reasoning could soothe her. We discovered through that social worker that Irene's pension, by itself, was just too large for meeting the means-test for getting any aid. And any means-tested government aid considered the entire household income, plus assets, anyway. We were well beyond that threshold in both income and assets. We were too productive in our lives to qualify for any government largesse.

In addition, in order to collect Social Security disability, a person must have contributed to Social Security for five of the last ten years. That was another main reason for officers to have part-time jobs in which they had Social Security deducted. Of course, as mentioned, Irene had not contributed since she joined the police force in 1990. The 6 percent pension contribution replaced Social Security benefits. After leaving the social worker and her explanations, and after my seeing Irene's concern, I became more determined.

Irene lightened the conversation on our way home and smiled, saying, "Don't worry, Tom. We can sell this car. That will pay for the nurse to say 'Good morning' at our next visit. You can drive me around in the other one. I always wanted to sit in the back and be chauffeured. Then we could sell all our furniture. That will pay for the nurse following up with, 'How are you?' No problem. There's always the house, my shoes and my right arm, too. We can handle that."

Irene added that she wasn't driving much at that time anyway. We laughed a little. We were followed along I-4 by the reflection of the cross on the domed building.

When Irene saw that bright image, she let out a big "Whoopee!"

That was only one of Irene's favorite exclamations. Another one was "Woo-woo," when she caught me in my shorts. She was always expressing those little terms of endearment while disregarding her own pain and discomfort. I hope I did the same.

Everything changed in just a few days, as Irene and I were driving along one of the main streets in a suburb of Orlando, looking for marquees advertising insurance. I decided to return to an insurance store we had visited a few weeks earlier when we were told about COBRA. The agent we spoke to at that time promised she would do more research. The world is a better place because of such client-oriented employees.

She liked Irene (to meet her is to love her) and commiserated with her because this lovely person had family who had passed away due to cancer. She greeted us, saying she was about to call us. She found two high-deductible plans mandated by Florida law. Blue Cross and United Health were the carriers this friendly woman could represent. There were provisions that she was sure Irene could meet, knowing Irene's past coverage.

The provisions, as we understood them, were as follows (but do your own homework; rules change):

1. A client must have had continuous coverage up to at least eighteen months in the past (Irene had been covered since 1990 right up to the present).
2. Premiums must have always been paid on time (the city paid the bills).
3. There was never any proof of falsification that caused a break in coverage (Irene passed that test).

Next question: how much? We were happy to cover the policy premium, deductibles, co-pays, co-insurance, and any additional "maximum out-of-pocket expense." We estimated that for Irene's coverage alone, it would be more than $20,000 a year, not counting several thousand dollars additional for prescriptions and not considering my premiums and prescriptions. That's still about one chemo session in Irene's case. There was a deadline to submit Irene's application.

We did the required research on Irene's past treatment, summarized it all up-to-date, and got it back to the agent the next day. That diligent agent faxed it to United Health, our preferred provider, after studying both policies.

The memo to the insurance company in early spring of 2011 included this final paragraph written by Irene. She lived for more than fourteen months after she wrote this paragraph.

My care has been very aggressive, and it has allowed me to beat the odds to this time. For that, I am very grateful. Among the horrid times, in which cancer has been part of my life during the past seven and a half years, there were some very happy and decent periods of normalcy—and I'm praying there will be more.

Next—prescription coverage. The same company also offered a prescriptions plan. Irene was taking some extremely expensive meds, some top-tier level with the most expensive co-pays. We'd handle it.

We were not absolutely certain of the new coverage until well into May. It was a nail-biter for a while. Irene still had chemo appointments in April and May.

Irene was finally accepted. We became, once again, focused on Irene's care and course of treatment. We were very happy to pay whatever it cost. Irene was delighted and exhilarated. That was the way I liked to see her—smiling. Her tears crushed me. She no longer had a guilty conscience, though there was never a need for her to feel that way. We direct-deposited the premiums for the next year and twenty-two days, from June 1, 2011, until Irene passed on June 22, 2012. We ensured all other expenses were paid immediately. We did not want to risk being dropped.

Irene and I both thanked God that our dilemma ultimately was resolved. At times, we heard someone say that we were lucky to be able to get the best care available for Irene—many can't afford it. We know that, and we sympathize. We are happy we made some right choices in life.

It wasn't luck that enabled us to work through the financial hazards the cancer diagnosis presented. It was preparing for many years and trying to make sure things fell into place. No, it wasn't luck at all that Irene and I could afford our insurance coverage in retirement. I hope you have done some preparation too. It certainly enhances the quality of life during the course of treatment.

Keep in mind that finances are always on the minds of most patients going through cancer treatments. Fortunately, for Irene and me, it worked out, after considerable anxiety.

"It's a good thing we were able to get coverage, Tom. Did the cross have anything to do with it?"

"I don't know, honey, but houses are cheap up north now. We could have still kept this house and bought another one up there."

"I didn't want to have to move up there again, Tom. I want to stay right here with you."

"You're right, honey. I don't feel like it either. I thank God and the cross, I guess, that we got the coverage. Otherwise, I would have had to chauffer you around if we sold one of the cars."

A smiling Irene snickered at my tongue-in-cheek referral to subservience. "You do that anyway, sweetheart. We don't need to waste any time on another move. We need each other and every last moment we have left—and who knows how long that will be?"

Treatment Continued

Irene gained six pounds in between visits. We were all glad about that. It strengthened her to contend better with the infusions. Chemotherapy had been discontinued until healing of the internal stomach fistulas could take place. That precaution seems to have worked. Irene was eating more and becoming less and less dependent on the tube feedings. The oncologist decided it was time to restart the chemo infusions, considering the worsening of Irene's disease during the delay. Chemo was resumed at reduced levels.

Since October 6, 2010, Irene had the enteral feeding tube through her intestine for nutrition. It caused us many problems and was replaced a total of five times but still remained very troublesome. It was last replaced at the end of March 2011, with the largest diameter size available, as I mentioned previously. Our next scheduled evaluation of the insertion site was on April 18, 2011. The surgeon who placed it wanted to inspect it, and Irene wanted to decide whether or not to remove it, once and for all.

04/18/2011: Surgeon says just a little while longer with this darn tube. She sees healing and drainage is less. I still have loose stools and fatigue. She says to reduce Jevity feeds and eat more (bananas, for example), so as to be as independent as possible from the tube. She'll pop over next week to GI clinic when I have my appointment for chemo and look at it again. I think she is tired of it too but wants to be cautious.—I. C.

The problem with the feeding tube and the insertion site continued. Irene's negative reaction to the infusions relentlessly continued, but she was handling it all with her usual grace and pleasant smiles. I knew how much she was hurting, both physically and emotionally, but I don't think many others did. It was painful to witness this beautiful and delightful woman suffering so much. She hid her discomfort from the rest of the population.

04/26/2011: Chemo with irinotecan and Erbitux continues. The plan will be to continue chemo every two weeks and have CAT scans every month to watch the effectiveness. My latest scans were not encouraging. Regular side effects; they never stop.—I. C.

Earlier in the year, the oncologist prescribed a tiny dose of tincture of opium to alleviate the diarrhea. I administered it once, at that time, through the main feed-line Y junction. Irene had shortness of breath almost immediately. That one dose did help with the diarrhea though. The oncology PA suggested it again, but when we told her of Irene's trouble breathing, the PA said to stay away from the opium. The standard bananas-and-rice regimen was again proffered.

05/10/2011: Same cocktail. Nodules stable. We won't have to move back up North. We have insurance coverage. A lot more expensive than what it used to cost.—I. C.

Irene could not shake the overwhelming fatigue. Driving to Bradenton to visit Maria was quite an effort, but she wanted to do it. Now and then on our return trip to Orlando, we would detour. There was Plant City, which offered us the strawberry shortcake, and that little tearoom near Lake Alfred that provided a little relaxation and diversion from the grinding routine of chemo sessions. Lakeland was interesting too. We also had something to look forward to at our next appointment:

05/24/2011: Success. The surgeon who placed the tube said the tube was causing more discomfort than benefit. The surgeon was very happy to remove it for me. I am eating enough and put on more weight. Tom hasn't had to hook me up for a while. Surgeon said she thinks the insertion site wound would heal within two weeks. I hope so. What a relief. I feel better already. I feel normal. Tom will keep it clean and put an ostomy bag over it until it heals.—I. C.

I commented, "That was simple. I could have done that and saved us a trip."

We all laughed a little. Each of us was very happy to be done with all the trouble that darn tube had caused us over the last eight months. But in the end it did the job. Irene was gaining weight and after a while, the wounds healed. They left a couple more ugly scars on Irene's tummy, but that was a small price to pay to be rid of it. At last, Irene was unencumbered by any tube or pump. It freed us to quite an extent. Liberation! Quality of life vastly improved. A battle was won but not the war.

We celebrated on occasion by meeting my sister and brother-in-law for dinner at a seafood restaurant. That was a terrific treat. Imagine, Irene and I going out to din-din. That hadn't happened very often recently. It made Irene feel human again. It is a pleasure many people—and couples—take for granted. Think about that the next time you and yours are in a nice restaurant. The couple in the next booth may be celebrating the removal of a feeding tube. If they are, I'll bet they will be holding hands across the table. If they aren't, they should be.

Although Irene and I did not know it at the time, by the end of May 2011, she would have just a little over a year left in her too-short and troubled life. Neither of us knew she also had completed her 164th normal chemo infusion.

By the end of June, there was only a little bit of drainage coming from the insertion site. It was almost healed, but I still had to keep an ostomy bag secured over the wound to prevent soiling of Irene's clothes. I had to clean it regularly and apply balm to prevent the acidic yellowish fluid, which occasionally still leaked around the site, from burning Irene's skin.

By the end of July, Irene completed her 168th infusion, still with the irinotecan and Erbitux cocktail, plus Avastin. Her side effects lasted at least five full days after each session. Her sore lips, mouth, and tongue were problematic, along with the usual nausea, vomiting, and diarrhea. Over-the-counter remedies as simple as Chap Stick and Anbesol were often useful. She handled the symptoms bravely.

In the morning, Irene and I would lounge on the lanai with "cawfee" and watch the unending variety of sunrises. At least once, a shuttle launched from Cape Canaveral while we watched. The Cape is an hour's drive from our home. We watched the fireball and its white exhaust trail as it climbed into the early-morning heavens. We heard the sonic boom that rattled our windows when shuttles returned to the Cape. There were other launches of smaller payloads we occasionally watched, if they were in the mornings.

My sister and brother-in-law and sometimes one of my nieces called to see if they could visit. Irene was always up for company at this time. My family would connect us to the outside world, but our pace was noticeably slowing during the summer of 2011. I think everyone began to sense it.

By August 30, Irene had her 171st chemo session, after the usual unit of magnesium and other medications to relax her. The appointments, including blood draws, scans, meeting with the oncologist team, and finally, the infusion itself, occupied a full day at the hospital, not including the travel time. We had gone through that routine both at Fox Chase CC and Moffitt CC for eight years by this time, ever since August 2003. During that time, most other people's lives continued normally but not our lives. We reflected on the previous eight years and simply hugged each other, knowing that it was *our* battle to fight.

09/14/2011: Disappointing scans. The cancer is progressing. All the nodules are larger. Oncologist is recommending FOLFOX again. Oxaliplatin did the best against my cancer, but it had the worst side effects. But I think it's critical that we slow down the growth of the nodules. FOLFOX can do it if I can handle it without going into a reaction like before. Team said they did the research and could not confirm that I was allergic to it, just that I did have the severe side effects. They said if I am willing to undergo the side effects, they might be able to desensitize me to it by lowering the dose and infusing it over twelve hours. They emphasized that the irinotecan and Erbitux is not effective anymore. They said they could try a few sessions of FOLFOX at normal dosage first and watch me closely and then do the scans. They would give me potent pre- and post-medications to help with the side effects. I told them I would do it. I want to continue chemo. They were glad to hear me say that. So was Tom. They will confirm the plan by next chemo session in two weeks, 09/27.—I. C.

Irene finished her 172nd infusion in mid-September, knowing that future side effects would be horrible. She was both apprehensive and eager, however, to do whatever it took to defeat or delay this horrible disease growing inside her.

09/27/2011: Decision made. Skipped scheduled chemo today to get stronger for FOLFOX to start next week, 10/04.—I. C.

10/04/2011: Had my first FOLFOX in a while. So far, with all the pre-meds, the skipping last week's chemo, and everything else, side effects not too bad. I expected worse. It does tire me out, though. I can't wait to see scans after the next infusion. Hope they show improvement and that I continue to handle the oxaliplatin.—I. C.

Irene received her second dose of FOLFOX, her 174th infusion, two weeks later on October 18. She had a bad reaction: serious shortness of breath, red flushing of her face and ears, and tingling and numbness in her hands and feet—the same side effects she'd had a few years ago. They discontinued oxaliplatin with this particular session but continued the infusion with the 5-FU and leucovorin, the other two components of the FOLFOX cocktail, plus the Avastin.

11/02/2011: Tom and I arrived at the hospital by 7:00 AM to start twelve hours of my desensitization to oxaliplatin, the most potent drug against my disease and the only effective one left. I have had every normal chemo protocol. Unfortunately, after about four hours, I couldn't breathe. They had a "stat" emergency for me. They resuscitated me with oxygen and other injections. That was the end of oxaliplatin and any other normal chemotherapy regimen. I cannot be "challenged" with it any more. And nothing else is effective.—I. C.

In early November, Irene received her 175th and last *normal* chemotherapy. Any other protocol, from now on, would be conducted by the Clinical Research Unit (CRU). We were entering into another major phase of Irene's treatment—no more surgery; no more *normal* chemotherapy.

After all her many hospital admissions, Irene went from not qualifying for any additional surgery, after six majors, to not being eligible for any other normal chemo that was appropriate for Irene's colon cancer, after 175 of them. She had immunotherapy, radio-embolization, stent insertion and reinsertion, and a few other shorter procedures (for example, the Greenfield), and more than five tube replacements, plus the red ones. Irene also suffered a year of external feeding. We ordinarily informed our families after each one of the major stumbling blocks. We did the same this time. Of course, everyone was disappointed, along with us.

We kept two more appointments by the end of the year, both to discuss Irene's eligibility for participation in clinical trials. On the last one, December 14, a specific trial was mentioned, but the GI team wasn't sure when it would start. The team was searching their databases and hearts to find something that could give Irene hope. It might have been that they wanted her to be able to clutch onto something—anything—to get her through the Christmas holidays. It was not a very celebratory season for us this time. It was to be our last Christmas together, but we didn't know that.

Nevertheless, we traveled to Bradenton. There were two whole turkeys for the gang. Irene and her sister agreed that one of the turkeys was of better quality—before they were cooked—than the other, and it showed in the after-cooked tasting. The discussion regarding the quality of each turkey seemed very unimportant to me, considering what was going on in our lives. But it was important to Irene and Tammy. They were hoping the birds would taste good after cooking. They wanted the guests to enjoy them. In reflection, I think it was a good thing. To me, portions from both the turkeys tasted fine.

Irene and I had our last "private" dance together in the foyer of her sister's home. Irene's sister snapped a photo of us, embracing, doing a slow dance to "White Christmas." There we were, in sunny Florida, dancing to a tune while we imagined snow. I have misplaced that photo, I am very sorry to say. I should have framed it.

While we held hands in slow-dance fashion, we kibitzed a bit, back and forth:

"You're leading me, honey," I said.

"No, I'm not. You're leading me!"

Out of the corner of my eye I saw Tammy grab a camera and take aim. I attempted to get Irene to stop dancing and hold still.

"Let's just stay still for a minute, honey."

"Hey! I just saw a flash go off. That was my sister." Irene smiled broadly.

"We should have been kissing, honey. Give me my Christmas kiss."

"Love you, handsome."

"Ditto, beautiful. We should go over to Disney's Boardwalk to that dance hall. After dancing, we can go to the craft beer place for their sampler. Then we could watch the fireworks coming from Epcot. We've had that sampler before with Tommy and Chris, but we haven't danced over there, honey."

"Let's do it, Tom, tomorrow night."

A Different Path Ahead

Due to the severe reaction Irene had in November 2011 to her last dose of chemotherapy, even though it was administered over a longer period, the medical team came to the scary conclusion that Irene would not be able to receive any more normal, or standard, cocktails. For more than eight years, Irene's body had tolerated the severe trauma of surgeries and infusions. But the heroic struggle had taken its toll on her now-very-weary body.

About a year or so ago, we were told there would be no more surgeries. And now, there would be no more normal chemotherapy. So 2012 left us with no option, other than clinical research trials. Psychologically, that put us into a different frame of mind. We'd run out of the standard treatment regimens. It was momentous for us. Maybe it was a mountain too high.

Our GI oncologist, therefore, made the referral to the Clinical Research Unit on the second floor of the same building. An appointment for February 2 was confirmed. An enrollment process determined a patient's eligibility for one of the clinical trials currently being performed at Moffitt. It was a strict screening process because results of studies at various stages had to be controlled in order to validate the findings.

02/02/2012 AM: Our first visit to CRU. Scans and blood work for baselines. I hope Tom and I get an extension on life. I'm getting scared. No more surgery; no more regular chemo. We want quantity.—I. C.

Irene had applied for nonstandard protocols in the past, upon the recommendation of the medical team. Remember the leukapheresis trial? The strict requirement was that the candidate had to have had colon cancer that metastasized to the liver and must have had a liver surgery to remove it. Finally, the patient's scans must not have revealed any hypermetabolic activity anywhere. The drug being tested, if effective, would prevent the return of cancer to the liver. Irene had qualified, but her cancer returned. That was one of many disappointments we faced through the years.

The therasphere process was also a very recently approved Moffitt procedure for colon cancer that metastasized to the liver. It was not only unsuccessful for Irene but caused quite a bit of discomfort for her afterward, to put it mildly. Irene had to get nutrition externally. Cancer treatment is a long way from being perfect, but the effort continues. Researchers need patients to participate in nonstandard solutions to finding a cure.

When we were first assigned to those particular trials, we had some confusion regarding certain phraseology that the medical staff used in their everyday conversations. Everyone undergoing cancer therapy should go to official websites such as Cancer.gov (the National Cancer Institute's homepage). Internet search engines (such as Google) can aid in that search. Official websites provide accurate information and can help you understand the myriad of medical terms.

In late 2011, we were told that samples of Irene's liver cancer cells would be sent to Ireland to see if she would qualify for a Phase II trial that Moffitt's CRU was involved in. Irene didn't qualify—wrong kind of cancer cells.

Another time we were told that her liver tissue was sent to Germany (Bayer Health) for a Phase III trial. I'm not sure of the specifics of the phases of the trials for which Irene did *not* qualify, because the records are proprietary, and Irene was not an actual participant—only her liver and colon cancer cells were.

We basically went along for the ride at that time, our heads spinning.

"We're getting down to the wire, Tom."

"Yes. But we're not there yet. Hang in there, Irene."

"I will, Tom, as long as you're beside me."

"I am, honey. I'm here."

Chapter Ten

Clinical Research Unit: First Attempt

Irene eventually qualified for a Phase I clinical trial. After a few false starts, Irene was finally accepted into "MCC15267, a Phase I clinical trial utilizing 1-methyl-D-tryptophan in patients with advanced malignancies." We were confused—what did it all mean regarding Irene's cancer?

Note that in all trials, any participant can leave the study whenever he or she chooses and for whatever reason; for example, bad side effects.

The distinction between experimental trials, clinical trials, and standard treatment regimens needs clarification. Important differences separate them. The various phases (Phase I, II, III, or IV) were Greek to us—we had only a vague idea of the differences between these terms. We were very befuddled at first.

Experimental trials claim to be better or to replace conventional or standard cancer treatments. One major difference between experimental trials and clinical trials is that the latter has advanced to FDA-approved *human* participation. Petri dishes, Bunsen burners, and animals are important in such progress—don't take me wrong. They are a long way, however, from a cure.

The proponents of experimental treatments hold out hope for people who have usually run out of other standard methods, such as the usual surgery, radiation, chemotherapy, and immunotherapy. Experimental trials put in place theoretical protocols. Some patients, maybe movie stars, try experimental treatment from the very beginning of their diagnosis, even though it is controversial and unproven. Or they may do it later. They may go overseas, where the trial has been approved in certain countries. Experimental remedies are not widely available and are not usually covered by regular insurance policies.

Experimental trials are conducted in US university research centers and other institutions around the country and elsewhere and are probing new treatments all the time. Funding comes from government and charitable grants. Private companies are also in the race to find cures and methods to improve both quantity and quality of life for cancer patients.

I recently heard that a coordinated effort will be attempted. Focus, such as the NASA mission to land astronauts on the moon by the end of the '60s, may be fruitful with the proper leadership and funding to accomplish it. I read that one of the societies pushing for that concentration of effort is known as the Super Bowl of cancer professionals, the American Society of Clinical Oncology. Let's keep hoping and praying.

Also in the future, maybe gene therapy, nanotherapy, and other protocols still in their incubation stages will be part of the standard treatments. But right now they have to go through several screens in order to be tried by research institutions. Plenty of legal, ethical, and social parameters must be considered. The FDA, National Institutes of Health, and at least two scientific institutions, according to the established rules, all have to approve or recommend any research or use of an experimental therapy. That all makes them pretty scarce and unavailable to most cancer patients, for the time being.

Clinical trials usually come in four phases: I, II, III, and IV. Each phase has its specific purpose and very strict requirements for patients to enroll in each.

Phase I clinical trials are searching for a safe dosage and how it should be administered: orally (pills); intravenously (injection); or, systemically (port).

Phase II trials, after completing Phase I purposes, have the objective of determining if the new drug affects the specific cancer cells under study. Phase II also continues studying any effect on the human beings participating in the trial.

Phase III trials, having gone through I and II segments, advance the research even further. They compare the new regimen to current standard treatments. There's a good idea of dosage, affect, and side effects. The new drug shows promise by this phase.

Phase IV trials continue to assess the long-term effectiveness and safety of the new drug, while firming up the results of the first three phases. Phase IV trials have advanced farther along toward improvement in treatment than the first three phases. It's the best one to be involved in. It often takes many years to go from a Phase I to a Phase IV trial.

The purpose of any clinical trial and establishing its objectives involves several elements. Of course, the actual reason for the trial has to be clearly stated. Who can participate and how many people are needed in the sample of participants has to be determined, so that the study has validity and the results are not happenstance or coincidental. The amount and frequency of use by the patient of any other drugs or prescriptions has to be strictly controlled and documented.

No other remedies of any kind can be used simultaneously—that could distort findings and cloud actual results. Which remedy was a success or which one failed? Did the additional remedy support or deteriorate the effectiveness of the new drug? Before Irene could join a study, there was a window that had to be established since her last standard treatment. Isolation of the trial's findings is absolutely required. When undergoing a clinical trial, no other kinds of external therapeutic methods are allowed.

To further protect the trial against faulty or unsubstantiated data, the administrators have to establish which medical and diagnostic tests should be performed and how often. Initial blood tests and scans can determine baselines for measuring growth, diminishment, or disappearance of tumors. But those tests have to be timely and ongoing to firmly monitor results of the study.

The actual gathering and compiling of all the information learned is necessary too. That often takes a lot of coordination from many locations around the country, from several hospitals and research centers. Remember the Phase III study Irene had high hopes for? It had seventy-two participants from around the country. Only twelve of them were from Moffitt Cancer Center.

Besides being in a certain age group to be involved in that study, Irene had to have the very specific type and stage of cancer. As I previously mentioned, she had to have already had very certain kinds of treatments and symptoms to be included in that Phase III trial: colon cancer metastasized to her liver; a liver resection; and no discernible disease shown on scans after her liver surgery. Irene was elated when we got those scan results, and she qualified for that very promising study.

But in her case, the cancer returned. That study involved a control group and a placebo. That's the normal procedure in Phase III studies. Irene either had the placebo, or the new drug did not have the desired effect in her case. The administrators never tell the patient or their doctors who has the placebo and who has the new drug. In Phase III trials, the patient never knows whether he or she was in a random or control group.

On February 2, 2012, Irene and I reported to our first appointment at the CRU on the second floor to apply for possible enrollment in a Phase I trial. We wished it was a Phase IV, but at this juncture, we had to take what was available. It was better than nothing at all. The appointment had to have a window of at least twenty-eight days *after* any kind of standard treatment. It was a few weeks before Christmas when Irene had her last treatment. We were home for the holidays.

We really hoped for miracles or a brand-new FDA-approved drug that was a cure and immediately available. Maybe on our drive to Moffitt we'd hear the news bulletin come through on my smartphone. Come to think of it, that would be a miracle, wouldn't it?

Remember that dome-shaped storage facility constructed of some kind of shiny material where we always saw the reflection of a cross? It was halfway to and from Moffitt on the north side of Interstate 4. We eagerly looked for it on every trip, hoping to see it again. We were looking to be comforted.

On that first day at the CRU, Irene had to get the baseline scans and urine and blood tests. That morning she still had the persistent pain in her abdomen, the normal fatigue that plagues all cancer patients, and the constant nausea. Besides the headaches, night sweats, lack of appetite, and diarrhea, all of which she adapted to, she wasn't complaining; she was just very nervous and hoping to survive. She looked very pretty in her pageboy hairstyle and light-blue sweater. That was my favorite color on her. She smiled and said she'd worn it for me, to brighten my day. Irene was always thinking of me, not herself, even in those mentally dreary days.

After the scans and blood tests, we were interviewed by an advanced registered nurse practitioner (ARNP), a nurse with a very advanced degree and a specialty in oncology on top of that.

A full history of past and present illness, fistulas, surgeries, stent replacements, prescription usage, allergies, social history, family situation, and every other parameter regarding health and other matters over Irene's entire life were covered. It was an extensive interview process—necessarily. The initial report I later read was thorough and impressive. With its preformatted headings, it reminded me of an official Philly Police Department homicide investigation report from my old days as a detective. It followed a predetermined format with sections and subsections to be completed by the investigator, or the ARNP, in this case.

There were pages and pages of information. Even the backrubs and massages I gave Irene, when she spent too many days in bed and got muscle-sore, were recorded in the interview.

After the intake interview, we anxiously waited in a CRU anteroom until the scan results were available.

In a couple of hours, we got the results of the scans and blood and urine tests. It was a shock. We had expected a little worsening over the break. The scans were, however, lit up with spots and nodules throughout Irene's whole midsection and lungs. A lot had happened over the holidays. The tumor in her liver now measured about 2¼ x 2½ inches, much increased since the last scans. It was depressing. We held hands as we got the news. Irene and I could not prevent the tears.

02/02/2012 PM: Scans show extensive spreading! How could so much cancer grow so fast?—I. C.

I can't imagine what went through the mind of that ARNP who delivered that scan report to us. She was very definitely affected by telling us. She offered tissues that were on her desk. I'm sure it wasn't the first time for her.

I had flashbacks to my assignment in Homicide in the 1970s. There were times when I had to tell parents that their teenage or twenty something child had been murdered. That was the worst part of the job. I always dreaded that part of my duties.

We were losing the battle. Irene had a lot to overcome and had only the possibility of a Phase I trial to aid in her recovery. We girded for whatever the next step was to be.

Preliminarily, Irene was accepted and enrolled in the trial. The initial step was taken and accomplished—qualification. But how helpful can a Phase I trial be? We were told to come back to the CRU on February 7, 2012. It would be a very long five-day intermission.

02/02/2012: On our way home from CRU, the sign of the cross was brilliant. Was it a message? And what was the message? I wonder what the side effects of the pills will be. Tom is very quiet.—I. C.

During the entire time until the next appointment, Irene was conscious every moment of continued growth and spreading of the disease within her body.

"Tom. Look how big the lump on my stomach is getting. It hurts to touch it."

"Yes, I see, honey. Try not to touch it."

It was very personal for her. We each felt the apprehension welling up in the other. In quiet moments later that week, we began speaking in more detail of what Irene's wishes were regarding funeral arrangements. When the doctors told us there would be no more surgeries a year ago, we discussed cremation and told her family about it. We'd known for years that we wanted cremation instead of burial. We thought it was wise to inform her family again—and mine too.

Moving on to more pleasant thoughts, Valentine's Day was close to two weeks away. Could we have a mini-celebration at home, maybe with Pat and Don? We needed some comforting company. My sister and Don were great listeners. We didn't constantly hear about their own aches and pains, though they had them. They lived close by and always were ready to visit. If Irene was up to it, maybe we could go to Bonefish seafood restaurant. "That would be nice" was a recurring expression of Irene's. Whenever I suggested an outing or dinner or the movies, her response was almost always, "That would be nice," except toward the end, when she was bedridden most of the time. If I asked if she wanted tea or toast, though, she used that response, as long as she had the breath and strength to form the words.

We were told that the delivery of the drug in the upcoming clinical trial was neither intravenous nor systemic. It required Irene to take ten large pills in the morning and ten more in the evening. The pills couldn't be crushed, either. Even though it concerned Irene whether she would be able to swallow the pills, it was better than infusion. Oral intake was more liberating; it could be done at home. One of the nurses assigned to the CRU suggested taking fluids through a straw when Irene was swallowing the large pills. Later, she tried that, and it did make the lengthy process of ten pills at a sitting go much smoother. It was a very good and practical tip. Would it really matter in the long run?

Irene was reciting her rosary and novenas to herself, all the way to the hospital and on the return trip home. I saw the rosary beads and holy card in her hands. She looked peaceful on the outside, curled up on the reclined passenger seat. I didn't want to interrupt her thoughts and prayers.

In our bedroom on her night table, rosary beads hung from the lampshade. A St. Theresa of the Roses novena holy card was always nearby too. The night table's bottom drawer contained short prayer books and a liturgical missal I found in my own belongings, when Irene asked for one a couple of years ago. The top drawer held all her prescriptions that didn't fit on the table top because of tissue boxes, a constant bottle of Gatorade with straw, the lamp, and the most frequently used pill containers that needed to be handy. If Irene wanted my help, I gave her a little brass bell she could shake if I was in another room—she couldn't raise her voice loud enough for me to hear her faint call. I picked it up at a flea market years earlier. I'd kept it as an ornament on my office desk. It finally came in handy.

We wanted and needed the company of loved ones. Irene's family would make the two-and-a-half-hour drive and bring several frozen containers of soup we could defrost over many days.

Pat and Don also called at the perfect time. I asked them to come over and visit. They said they would come over the very next day with some refreshments, something easy for Irene to eat and something hardier for me. I was losing a lot of weight, too. When Irene didn't eat, I didn't eat.

Next day, Pat and Don arrived with arms full of plastic containers and ceramic bowls. My favorite supper dish in the whole world is what my siblings and parents called "the old reliable." When other ingredients were not plentiful, we could always rely on my mother's mixing up inexpensive ground beef, onions, and gravy. Alongside that staple she always included mashed potatoes. We kids used a piece of bread with butter to scoop up into our hungry mouths our own personal and individual amount of potatoes and meat, with onions and gravy.

The old reliable remains my favorite dinner to this day. It's something like Shepherd's Pie, but in most restaurants the ratio between the meat and potatoes is not my personal choice—too much mashed potatoes; not enough meat and gravy. The restaurant version doesn't lend itself to scooping either, especially in a public atmosphere. Pat and Don brought enough of the old reliable to last me for several days with just microwaving.

For Irene, they brought homemade chicken with rice soup, one of Irene's favorites. To top off the meals they brought some "Butterscotch Krimpets" and small, snack-sized pies from a bakery in Philadelphia, Tastykake. The company only recently had expanded distribution into the Orlando area. They were a special treat when we could find them for sale. The fast-food chain, Wawa, carried them.

The array of familiar food hit the spot. We could, over our meal, talk of the old days and make comparisons to the Ukrainian and Irish upbringings. For example, Pat's high school days were spent at Little Flower High School for Girls in Philadelphia. St. Theresa of the Roses, one of Irene's patron saints, was also the school's patroness. She was known as "the Little Flower" in the Catholic religion. It was a coincidence from which we all derived some comfort. Some of you may remember the hit song, "St. Theresa of the Roses," from 1956. That was before it became politically incorrect for artists to express their faith, if they have one today.

The intervention of St. Theresa was invoked during serious illnesses by petitioners and their loved ones. If the Little Flower "heard" the plea for intercession, she would send a rose or roses as a sign of acknowledgment. Any rose sign satisfied Irene and others that the request was heard by the Little Flower. What was the danger in such prayer if it gave peace and comfort? None at all that I could think of. Of course, we always depended on our doctors, too.

My sister and her husband attended mass almost every Sunday. They jokingly claimed a 95 percent attendance record. They were far from being holy-rollers, but they were sincere, and their beliefs were personal—the same as Irene's and my own. We lived our lives accordingly. We all knew that about each other, and Irene appreciated that during their visits.

Both the spiritual and practical conversations removed us from the present, so we drifted into the more carefree and safe past. It was what the doctor ordered. We always depended on Pat and Don to bring some mirth and congeniality into our home. It abounded in their home, too.

Two days later, Pat and Don came over again. Their visits always uplifted Irene and me. Irene looked forward to the light talk and joviality. We got through most of that anxious period in relatively high spirits.

We had the appointment at CRU on Monday, February 7. But then, the previous Saturday night, February 5, Irene had a high fever. With aspirin and plenty of fluids, it diminished by Sunday morning. But as Irene was dressing, we both noticed that her skin was off-color. Jaundice? We had been here before. We noticed the slight change in hue in the master bathroom. It has a lot of natural light. The whites of her eyes looked normal, but we both got somewhat worried. The next day we would be in a hospital setting at Moffitt, but should we go to the local ER in the meantime? Irene refused that option with an emphatic, "No, thanks!" We'd wait until we got to Moffitt next day.

By Monday morning it was more obvious—Irene was at least a bit jaundiced. She felt very weak, too. In a couple hours we were supposed to start day 1, cycle 1 of the Phase I clinical trial. By this time, we were very worried.

On each visit to the CRU, there was always a brief interview by nurses' aides and a weigh-in. Irene's temperature and blood pressure were also measured. We didn't get far along the process before the ARNP spotted Irene and immediately sat us down in her office. It was very obvious by this time that Irene was fully jaundiced. She was feeling extremely weak and was running a higher temperature. Her blood pressure reading was dangerously low. The ARNP notified our oncologist, who right away admitted Irene to the Intensive Care Unit in the same building. There would be no starting the clinical trial today. Disappointment again!

That day was the first day of something else, though: a weeklong hospital stay in ICU. This was Irene's last hospital stay of her life. She was tremendously sick with cholangitis and other possible strange-sounding maladies. I knew that the suffix "-itis" meant inflammation and/or infection. At the time, I had no idea what "cholang-" indicated.

02/07/2012: Admitted to hospital today. I'm yellow. They suspect that the stent they put in me a year and a half ago might be blocked up. It wasn't as long-lasting as expected. Dangerous! At least I didn't have to go to the local ER. Thank God and St. Theresa for that. It's a good thing we had the appointment today to start the Phase I trial.—I. C.

When we knew Irene was to be admitted to the hospital, Irene sent me on an errand to retrieve hospital clothes from home. I made a list on my smartphone. I had to get the right stuff. I didn't want to just bring any old thing back to her. I made the three-hour round trip. My cargo included her "new pink robe, the pajamas from the middle drawer from the dresser next to the bedroom door, the pajamas hanging closest in the master bedroom closet, the pink-and-white slippers, toothpaste and toothbrush, shampoo, and four panties." Irene thanked me, as usual.

When Irene was hospitalized in the past, sometimes it was on short notice, like this time. I would run my errand. Other times, we knew ahead of time there would be an admission, and Irene had a small suitcase to bring along. Occasionally, I stayed over in the hospital and slept on a cot in Irene's room a few nights, if I had my toiletries and change of clothes with me. Sometimes, I made the round trip if the admission was unexpected.

Irene settled in and got ready for whatever was coming her way. The ARNP's medical report that prepped the floor doctors and nurses was well written, thorough, and quite longer than the usually tightly written condensed synopses of regular doctor's visits. It was as precise as the surgeons' reports I've read.

On the ICU floor of the hospital division at Moffitt, Irene was immediately started on "aggressive fluid resuscitation" intravenously. When the bevy of medical personnel surrounded her hospital bed asking questions, she told them she had significant pain, by this time, in her right upper abdominal quadrant (liver). She pointed to the big lump. She said the pain was like a huge rubber band squeezing and tightening on a regular basis.

When she told them what she was taking for the pain, they contacted the pain and palliative care doctor. Irene not only was taking a lot of Dilaudid, but she had two kinds of pain patches too. One was for her upper arm, and one I put directly on her abdomen, close to the painful bulge. The specialist told us how best to coordinate the use of the pain meds combination. We were using them "as needed," which was most of the time. That was not the best application of those narcotics. We needed better pain management.

As I recall, the purpose of the patches is ongoing pain relief over two or three days, when they would be replaced. The dilaudid was used as needed to "break through" pain that peaked. If followed, that application of pain medicine would probably better control it over longer periods, and each drug would be more effective. Regardless, Irene was always in constant pain to one degree or another. Who knows how severe the pain would have been without any meds? I can't imagine.

Cholangitis is a bacterial infection in the common bile duct. That duct is a tube, through which bile is dumped into the gall bladder and intestines, to help digest food. The bile is manufactured in the liver and sent through that bile duct down into the digestive system. Cholangitis can cause significant morbidity and mortality if untreated with antibiotics. In Irene's case, the medical staff were also concerned about sepsis, which is a potentially deadly blood-poisoning. Irene needed a procedure, that went by the acronym of ERCP, immediately.

About a year and a half before this attack, Irene had a stent—a tubular device to replace a duct or blood conduit—implanted during a surgical procedure. The stent probably needed to be exchanged regularly, anywhere from six months to a year. But we were so concerned with other details of Irene's cancer, we didn't remind anyone about replacing it. Besides, Irene's liver enzymes (bilirubin) were always normal in her numerous blood tests in the interim. There was no reason to suspect any blockage.

Scans revealed that the stent was seriously clogged. It needed to be exchanged with a new one immediately. The procedure that Irene would get the next day, February 8, after her admission to ICU, was as follows:

Irene (on a gurney) and I went to the suite on a different floor where the procedure would take place, and I asked the nurse for the actual name of the procedure Irene was undergoing—the ERCP. She made an attempt at pronouncing it. Giving up, she told me to wait a minute. Irene and I looked at each other, raised our eyebrows, and smiled. Irene knew what I was doing.

Abbreviated medical terms drive me crazy until I know what they mean. Then, I'd be the first to use the acronym, but using abbreviations when I don't know the meaning is pretentious. One time, after one of Irene's surgeries at Moffitt, our friendly surgeon told me I was high maintenance with all the questions I asked. She, of course, really didn't mind the questions at all. She liked both Irene and me—I think.

The nurse returned in a few minutes with a printout. With precise enunciation, the pretty nurse said, "If you must know, wise guy, it's called an endoscopic cholangiopancreatography. But I think that name doesn't include the 'R' in the abbreviation. The actual full name is probably even longer than endoscopic cholangiopancreatography. So there, Mr. Smarty-Pants!"

With a big smile, she handed me the four-page printout with diagrams and told me to memorize the contents by the time Irene's procedure was finished. She told me I had a little more than an hour, and I would be graded on my acquired knowledge. All three of us had a little laugh. We were all a little more lighthearted. Irene went into the surgery room with her usual happy smile. We kissed as she was rolled in. I told her I loved her. She voiced her love for me through her discomfort.

It was amazing! During the ERCP, the doctor and his helpers sedated Irene and wormed a device down her throat. The endoscope had little cutting tools and a camera on its tip. Organs were cut, stents were exchanged, and the whole area was protected against bleeding or infection—all guided and performed by viewing a monitor. That is, of course, a simplistic description of the procedure, but it suffices. All of that was accomplished without having to make an incision. All modern surgery is remarkable to me. I've seen a lot of it during the last nine years.

In about an hour, Irene was wheeled back to a recovery room, groggy, where I had been waiting and studying the four-page printout. The "R" in ERCP stands for retrograde, by the way. So the full name of the procedure is endoscopic retrograde cholangiopancreatography. I filled in the nurse, too. Now I could throw around that abbreviation whenever anyone asked me about that procedure. I still hope that if I do, any smarty-pants who asks me about it won't ask me to spell it. I'd have to refer to this paragraph.

Gradually, Irene became herself again. We kissed. We smiled. I was glad to have her back. She couldn't talk. Her throat was sore. But this hospital stay was just beginning. We were only in the second day of a total of seven days. There would be more worry and concern. Even though Irene was receiving antibiotics in big doses intravenously, by February 10, Irene's discomfort worsened after the ERCP.

02/10/2012: Really bad stomach pain. Severe nausea and vomiting. I can't eat anything. I don't want anything to eat. I just want the pain to go away. Hernia is still there, too.—I. C.

Irene was in agony after the stent exchange—throwing up and running a high fever for the next few days. The doctors suspected pancreatitis, not too uncommon after an ERCP. The scan also showed a "prominent loop of bowel" within the right upper abdominal quadrant, which concerned the team. There was a pocket of air and fluid there. There might be a digestive tract blockage, too.

Irene had been constipated since the procedure, on February 8, the day after she was admitted to the hospital. Prior to the exchange of stents, she had regular loose bowel movements. All of that contributed to Irene's pain. The antibiotics continued to flow through her body until finally, on February 13, the fever broke, the pain subsided, and we could think about going home—maybe the next day, St. Valentine's Day.

Through the many days of many hospital stays, Irene was visited by volunteer Catholic priests, Jewish rabbis, comfort dogs, musicians, and other good souls. On February 13, a female chaplain visited Irene. The reverend was making her rounds. I don't know what denomination she represented; she didn't say. During our three-way conversation, I asked the chaplain if she was aware of the legend of St. Theresa. Before she could answer, I began relating it. I didn't want to embarrass her. Being Protestant, she might not be current on Catholic saints.

I mentioned when I escorted her into the hall that I would surprise Irene with a dozen roses for the feast day when she got home the next day, but that gesture didn't count toward fulfilling the evidence of a "sign." The sign had to be inadvertent and not contrived. The reverend thought the story was quaint and if it was comforting, the belief had a positive purpose. I don't know what was actually going through her mind, but she humored us and wasn't critical at all.

02/14/2012: Going home. Feel okay. And a very happy Valentine's Day to all.—I. C.

Irene was pleased with the two dozen roses I had placed in our bedroom. She apologized, naturally, for not getting me anything.

"Oh, Irene, Irene, I don't need anything. I have you."

"I love you." She still apologized. Believe me—I didn't beat her. That's just the way she was.

On Valentine's Day, Irene got a phone call at home. It was the chaplain we'd just met the day before—the one I informed about St. Theresa of the Roses. I gave the phone to Irene.

"Guess what the woman's name is who took your bed after you left?" she asked Irene excitedly. "I'm with her now. Irene, her name is … Rose."

That is a true story! Irene and I looked at each other dumbfounded after she told me what the chaplain said. Irene told me that the chaplain was dumbfounded, too. I wondered what St. Theresa could do for Irene, now that we knew the saint had heard Irene's prayers? Irene's prayers were always personal. I wondered if the Little Flower could intervene in spiritual matters, if not in the physical world.

Clinical Research Unit: Second Attempt

On February 20, about a week after Irene was released from ICU, we were back at CRU. It was our second attempt to begin the Phase I trial. Irene still had persistent pain across her stomach. Irene had serious fatigue and some nausea without vomiting but very little appetite. She also had a mild temperature. She had lost some weight during the week. Irene went from 122 pounds, upon discharge from her last hospitalization, down to 111 pounds, a week later, at the weigh-in on February 20.

The only food I could get her to eat was a very chunky smoked fish spread I'd bought from a fresh-fish store that had opened recently over in St. Cloud. It was operated by a couple of young fishermen. They made the spread themselves. The proprietors knew Irene's story and made sure they always had enough for her. I spread it on rye toast. She really loved it, up to the last few weeks of her life, when she ate next to nothing. She ate the combo at least three times a day. She was getting some nutrition but not enough.

Irene's appearance changed dramatically. The ARNP's reports described Irene as a "delightful, thin, chronically ill-appearing female." Despite how Irene felt, she was still "delightful" in the ARNP's reports. Not too long ago, at our regular appointments with the physician's assistant in the GI suite, Irene was described as a "pleasant, well-groomed, and healthy-looking female." It seemed like Irene's decline was gaining speed and becoming apparent to others' eyes.

We were disappointed when the urinalysis performed as part of the standard intake routine was returned "cloudy," with a small amount of blood detectable. The white blood cell count was "too numerous to count," strongly indicating an infection.

Irene wouldn't be starting the Phase I trial that day. We began to worry about the twenty-eight-day screening process window for eligibility. It closed on March 1, and February was a short month. Irene had to be infection-free within nine days, or she would have to start all over again from the beginning. That would cost time. She was prescribed very strong medicine for a urinary infection, and I was told to get it filled at Moffitt's pharmacy, so Irene could start on it immediately—we weren't to wait until we returned home. Of course, I ran downstairs to the pharmacy, where I waited to have it filled. Irene took the first dose as soon as I returned with it.

We set up an appointment for another urinalysis in five days. At that time, finally, the test was negative. Next step—make the appointment to begin the trial and hope nothing prevented Irene from starting it. The date was set for February 28, just inside the eligibility window. It was another nail-biter.

Ongoing angst continued to plague Irene, as it does other cancer patients. The worries really never went away. Those few days between the first and second urinalyses were no exception, but we finally made it to the Phase I trial.

After that short delay, Irene started cycle 1, day 1 of the regimen: ten large pills in the morning and ten in the evening. By cycle 1, day 8, the urinary infection returned, causing another delay. She continued taking her thirteen prescriptions for nausea, pain, heartburn, blood thinning, constipation, appetite improvement, migraines, stomach soothing, and several others. Irene never stopped taking those, except that pills for constipation sometimes replaced pills for diarrhea.

Irene was able to continue in the trial through cycle 1, day 22, when we had another appointment on March 20. She proceeded through that week, which ended cycle 1. Irene was to return to CRU on March 27 to begin cycle 2, which lasted four weeks, just like cycle 1 had. After she completed that cycle, she would have the follow-up imaging scans and re-evaluation with our oncologist to assess her disease.

03/27/2012: Back in CRU. I'm very tired. My ankles have swelled for several days. Tom props my legs up all the time. I just want to sleep. I'm not hungry. Stomach hurts worse. Bulge in my abdomen is still getting bigger.—I. C.

Irene was supposed to start cycle 2, day 1 on March 27. Subsequent to the intake exam, the ARNP's report stated that "Ms. Cooney is a lovely 59 year old Caucasian female, who is unfortunately affected with metastatic colon cancer affecting her liver." The report also stated Irene was pale and drowsy but could be aroused easily. Irene's swollen ankles were noted too.

Neurologically, Irene had difficulty distinguishing sharp versus dull when the ARNP pricked her lower extremities. A blood test showed her hemoglobin was very low. She was anemic. She was transfused with a unit of packed red blood cells. She also received magnesium and potassium intravenously. We were given a prescription for magnesium with protein supplements, and I was told to sprinkle whey powder over her food. The ARNP increased the dosage of her upper arm patch, too. She could still proceed with the trial, taking the twenty pills at home every day, using a straw to help her get them down. We were sent home and told to return in two weeks, April 10, to continue the protocol.

04/08/2012: Still really tired. Can't get out of bed much. Got doctor in GI clinic to increase my Dilaudid and fentanyl patch for this terrible pain. Pain is getting worse and worse. Tom gives me my blood thinner shot every day. Swelling in my ankles went down a little. Tom just keeps adjusting the pillows under my legs. I have a rash on my cheeks. Might be from a new facial cleaner I started. My skin is so dry.—I. C.

04/10/2012: I have very little energy. I can't get comfortable because I have to lie on my back so I can keep my legs propped up. Back to CRU for cycle 2, day 15 of the trial. There's a little possibility that another Phase II trial will become available.—I. C.

Irene lost a little more weight after having gained a little. She was about 112 pounds. Her potassium and magnesium were at acceptable levels, and the urinalysis was negative for telltale signs of infection. That cleared the path for Irene to start cycle 2, day 15 of the trial. The doctors believed all of her distress symptoms were associated with her disease, not the study drug. Irene finished the Phase I trial after this last twenty-eight-day cycle. The final restaging scans were scheduled for April 24. We would meet with the oncologist that same day for review of the latest images. There was a possibility Irene could start a Phase II trial drug.

04/24/2012: Finished cycle 2, day 28 of Phase I trial. Preliminary screening for a new Phase II trial today, weigh-in, and blood work. Pain is worse. Doctor prescribed Oxycontin, but it made me throw up. I didn't like it at all. Bulge in my abdomen is getting larger by the day. Doctors will schedule new baseline blood work and scans in a few weeks.—I. C.

The ARNP's report after Irene's evaluation on April 24 read: "Chronically ill, frail, and thin-appearing" female, but "alert" this time.

The latest scans showed the disease had crept over to her pancreas, the linings of the stomach area, and just about her whole midsection. The cancer was getting worse.

The Phase I trial did not diminish Irene's disease at all. The cancer was extensive and causing her greater pain as each day passed. During the preliminary physical exams, the ARNP usually felt the abdominal bulge that resulted from the liver tumor getting bigger and bigger. This time the bulge was too tender. Irene flinched when the nurse went near it. It was horrible to helplessly watch my honey deteriorating so rapidly. All we could do was wait for our next appointment with the oncologist in the GI clinic. We scheduled the new Phase II trial intake exam, restaging scans, and evaluation for May 25, beyond the required twenty-eight-day window. Maybe the Phase II trial would have a better result.

Irene's Last Day to Ever Drive

Think about being ill and being unable to drive. Quite an inconvenience, isn't it? Now think about never being able to drive again. You are either too incapacitated or too old. Age seventy-six, in Ireland, is too old to rent a car. Imagine—I still can write a book, slow jog, peruse the Internet, be a caregiver, and be active in other ways, but to some governments, I will be too old to drive shortly. It's a milestone in your life. Will you mark the occasion of your last time behind the wheel? What will that do to your sense of independence?

In the meantime, I had to have my esophagus ablated—that meant the bottom end of my esophagus had some bad cells that needed to be burned off. There was a 5 percent chance the ailment could turn into cancer. It was uncomfortable most of the time and annoying all the time. It came from having a bad stomach.

I still have the problem—and have had it for the last several years—and every now and then, I have to get treated. Usually, the area is examined through an endoscopic examination—down the throat. Before the ablation, or burning process, was available, a patient had to get an endoscopy every year and eventually, it would probably require surgery.

The ablation process usually must be done about three times, and the ailment, Barrett's disease, often is cleared up after three treatments. And that's the end of it. I was due for my first one on May 17. My next one was in August, and my final one, I hoped, was on December 27, 2012. They were about three or four months apart, depending when the doctor could schedule the suite at the hospital. I was sedated during the procedure, naturally.

Irene drove only rarely during the last year of her life. May 17, 2012, was her last time, five weeks before she passed away. I had that special kind of endoscopic outpatient procedure in which I was sedated and not permitted to drive home afterward. My plan was to drive myself over to the hospital; get the procedure; bluff my way downstairs, avoiding the wheelchair; and get to the parking lot to drive myself home.

Both Pat and Don were working on the morning of May 17, but if necessary, Pat would pick me up at the hospital when I was discharged, if I was unable to escape. I could get my car later. Pat could be there by 3:00 PM. Based on the first time, when I had a preliminary short procedure that simply collected biopsies to confirm I had Barrett's disease, that timing would be close to right. It became the plan.

Irene would not have any of that. What if I were done at 11:00 AM? No, she insisted that she would do the driving. I would drive over to the hospital, but she would return home and then pick me up when I called her. At the time, Irene had rarely been getting out of bed, let alone out of the house and driving. I could see she wanted to do something for me, maybe a last gesture expressing her love and concern for me. I was very afraid because of the prescriptions she was taking, especially the painkillers, but she pleaded and cried. What was going through her mind? I relented.

Irene brought a pink plastic basin with her in the car that she was given for her own trips home from hospital stays, in case she had to throw up. In her pajamas, she came into the hospital and stayed with me until I was taken into the operating room. For about an hour beforehand, Irene chitchatted with me and the nurse who was hooking me up to the anesthesia leads and the various monitors. All that time, she was nauseated. For a couple of minutes, she rushed as fast as she could to the restroom when she couldn't hold it back any longer.

I was in post-op and recovery after the procedure for a few hours. Irene returned to pick me up. When we pulled into the garage, I said, "Thank you." I hold that picture in my mind to this day of that gorgeous smile, even though her eyes were sad. Her face had thinned. She was not much more than about a hundred pounds and very weak during the final several months. Her existence would end slightly more than a month from that afternoon when she drove me home from the hospital.

I don't think I ever thanked her in the past for driving me anyplace, as was her habit to thank me when I drove. Does anyone other than Irene express gratitude to his or her spouse after being driven to and from Wal-Mart to get groceries … or to the doctor? I wish I had thanked Irene just for holding my hand when I reached for hers and for providing me the privilege of doing so.

When I thanked her on that last day she would ever drive a car, she seemed grateful to me for letting her do that one final favor for me. I think she knew she would never drive again. Tears are welling in my eyes as I write this. Irene's natural persona was so sunny, sweet, delicate, and delightful. No one would ever mistake her for the stereotypical cop. She was such a beautiful person, inside and out. I miss every thoughtful gesture of hers and every word she ever said to me. I miss the grace she displayed during every bit of discomfort and pain she suffered through all the years I knew her. I miss everything about her.

Reclusive and Reflecting

From the end of April through Memorial Day weekend, we stayed mostly at home, except for Irene's last drive, reflecting on our time together. We talked about our police careers and how we met, the egg salad sandwiches, and "interviews" with Maria. We spoke mostly about the last eight and a half years since her initial diagnosis in August 2003. We remembered how we'd hoped that the abdominal pain was just female trouble. Then the biopsies told a very different, terrible tale.

We reflected on the first surgery that took eighteen inches of Irene's colon—that was Chuckie, the mild-mannered surgeon who did such a good job that the cancer never returned to her colon. She spent nearly two weeks in the Intensive Care Unit at Nazareth Hospital after that one. We recalled meeting the team and the placing of the port at Fox Chase Cancer Center and the side effects of her first chemo infusion. We joked about her hair loss over the next several years and the resulting rabbit fur.

Our thoughts next went to the surgeon who removed the right lobe of her liver and hooked up that external arterial pump. We had high hopes after that surgery. That didn't last long, though: blood clots, the Greenfield filter, many infusions, and lung resection all followed within the next few years at Fox Chase CC.

We also reflected on the good times we had together. We took advantage whenever possible during treatment breaks to get as much out of life as possible, under the circumstances. Irene thanked me for taking her places she had not visited previously. She thanked me for loving her and taking care of her. I thanked her for coming into my life, too.

We mentally revisited our move to Florida in 2006 and how much she loved our home there. We made that trip with the staples still holding her together after the lung resection. We had a little laugh about that. The PA who removed them on our first appointment at Moffitt Cancer Center couldn't believe Irene made the trip still stapled up. The PA got to know us very well, though, and later, knowing Irene better, she *could* believe it. She was with us for the rest of Irene's life. We experienced the PA's entire pregnancy with her second child, a boy. We have pictures of baby and mom.

Another liver resection, stomach surgery, TPN, and a feeding tube placement were in Irene's future. Irene's worse complication resulted from the therasphere procedure. It caused the first external feeding Irene had to endure—total parenteral nutrition. That got me far more involved in nursing than I had been. Worse yet was placing that external feeding tube that caused more pain, discomfort, and aggravation than any of Irene's procedures or surgeries in the past. Recovery from each surgery only lasted a few weeks; the external feeding and its leakage lasted months and months. Irene finally said, "I want it out!" Irene wanted to forget about that feeding tube chapter. So did I.

About 175 normal infusions, probably more, filled the time between the operations during the last almost nine years, up to the present. A zillion scans and various other diagnostic tests and blood work also kept us occupied with visits to the doctors and hospitals. It all had been quite a trip.

But now, we suspected we were coming to the end of our journey. Though we still had hope in our hearts, our rational side kept bringing us back to reality. I have no idea what was going through the minds of friends and family. They were very busy, I'm sure, with their own daily problems and concerns. May 25 arrived, and we went to see the oncologist.

Irene's Last Appointment at Moffitt Cancer Center

We wouldn't be celebrating Memorial Day weekend with anyone. The following is Irene's last entry in our chronicle.

05/25/2012: Oncologist said there's no more that can be done for me. Are we finally there? Tom and I just held each other. They left us alone for a while in the appointment room. They provided a list of hospice care associations. The oncologist gives me three to six months of living left. God, please prepare Tom and me through to the end.—I. C.

On Friday, May 25, 2012, following diagnostic scans in the morning, our oncologist told us there was nothing else Moffitt Cancer Center could do for Irene. She did not qualify for the anticipated Phase II trial. We wondered what our friends and relatives were doing and thinking while we were getting that earth-shattering news. How do we tell them?

Our very emotional medical team referred us to a social worker, who gave us the names of four different hospice organizations. Hospice of the Comforter operated in our county, and I'd heard good things about them. The Moffitt social worker contacted them.

The arrangements for hospice were set in motion. We left the hospital, saying good-bye to our medical team. We could tell they were saddened. The valet attendant retrieved our car, not having any idea of the news we'd just received. No one knew what was in our minds. They had their own concerns. Maybe that attendant had final exams that last week of May. Everyone was in his or her own world.

It was a very solemn drive home. We looked for the cross reflecting on the domed building. At dusk on an overcast day, we could still see it, however faint.

I pointed it out to Irene. "There's our cross, honey. Give me your hand, please. I love you."

Irene was softly weeping while saying her novena. She reached over, tearfully, and clasped my outstretched hand and smiled.

"I'm so glad I had you with me during this whole journey, Tom. You can't possibly know how much I love you for that. Remember, I was going to take care of you. It didn't work out that way, though."

"I wanted to be with you, honey. I always want to be with you. We still have time. We have time."

The very next day, Saturday, the administrative nurse from Hospice of the Comforter was sitting on my leisure chair in our bedroom, conducting the initial interview.

⚜

Chapter Eleven

Arranging Hospice

As I understand the standard insurance policy provisions regarding hospice, a doctor must verify that a patient has six months or less to live; that is, that the illness is terminal. There is a difference between hospice and home health care, which does not have that terminal requirement. Home health care may be temporary and intermittent.

Hospice may be in the patient's home, as in our case, or in a health care facility. Both the duration and the level of care may be limited in each situation. My point is that everyone should get familiar with a policy to ensure no surprises pop up, in the event a loved one becomes ill.

By Saturday, May 26, 2012, the administrative nurse from Hospice of the Comforter was very well informed about Irene's past medical history. Moffitt forwarded all the material she needed. During the interview, Irene was very conversant and smiling while she answered every question. Irene was resigned to her situation and decided to not let it affect her persona in front of others. Someone who didn't know her would have thought that she was a charming, pretty, cheerful, fifty-nine-year-old woman who was temporarily confined to bed due to an acute illness.

The nurse gave us a loose-leaf binder describing the entire hospice protocol, including the names and numbers of all the team members. Our team was called Teal, a very pretty color and fitting for Florida and its ocean and Gulf waters. After providing all the necessary insurance information, the nurse asked if Irene wanted to sign a Do Not Resuscitate order. *Wow! Are we there so soon?* I wondered.

This was a very momentous decision. I asked, "What actually does that mean? What about very basic life-saving techniques, such as CPR?" *Nothing* is done to interfere with the natural process of dying, we were told. There are no tubes or any other medical effort that an ambulance or fire/rescue team normally conducts, as with accidents or heart attacks, for example.

Irene did not want to be artificially kept alive. She wanted to "die in peace." Neither one of us believed her end would come in just over twenty-seven days. That was a shock that reverberates until this day. I find myself still shaking my head in denial when I think of it. *She can't be gone. But she is!*

We were instructed not to call 911, because they have a tendency to ignore DNRs. It's their job to resuscitate, regardless. They don't want to be placed in that situation. Irene said she accepted those terms, but her signing would wait until the doctor visited. A doctor had to witness her signature. That wasn't a problem. Irene understood better than I did, at that time, what lay ahead of us. The tumors in her abdomen were growing. They were very large and protruding and painful.

The doctor witnessed Irene's signature a couple days later. I noticed that Irene's formerly neat and expansive signature had changed. It was a bit slanted upwardly and tighter. She named me as her health surrogate to make all health decisions in the event she was unable to do so. Any and all phone calls, including what is considered an emergency, would go through hospice, twenty-four hours a day. They would coordinate all activity related to Irene's condition.

The next day the lead nurse visited. She was a model of proficiency. I filled her in on many of the details of Irene's medical history. She then gave Irene a thorough baseline physical exam, including all vital signs. She checked Irene's supply of medications, especially the pain pills. She called our Publix pharmacy to replenish them. I picked them up later that day.

We already had a shower chair, but the lead nurse decided to order oxygen and a bedside commode, and she thought about ordering a hospital bed too. Irene was in our king-sized bed. The hospital bed would make it easier to position her during baths and sheet changes. It could be raised or lowered, and it's easier for the caregiver to negotiate its perimeters. The oxygen arrived the next day, Monday morning. The oxygen machine was easy for me to adjust and operate. It was delivered with two back-up tanks, too.

As time slipped by, the hospice chaplain called, and a reverend came the following week. We prayed together. A representative from the parish visited and administered Holy Communion to both of us. A jovial nurse's aide very efficiently bathed Irene and changed the sheets. All was going smoothly. That was a very big help to me.

For the next several visits, Irene became less able to interact with us but could manage a smile, if not a complete response to the nurse's questions. She was very sleepy. With the medications Irene was still able to take, including the pain patches, she was suffering less. I was told the natural process of dying was taking place. After two weeks of hospice, Irene had no appetite, even less than during the previous several months.

Irene's beautiful skin was drying, and I saw wrinkles on her previously flawless facial skin. The etchings were slowly becoming more pronounced over the past year. Up until then, her face was smooth. She'd lost a lot of weight. The gaunt hollow between her shoulders and breasts told the tale of the emaciation the horrid disease caused. Her arms were so very thin. All this I now noticed.

I refused to see the cosmetic changes over the previous months that indicated my honey was losing her life. She was still beautiful to me. But the changes forced themselves into my mind. I didn't want to accept it, any of it. Her appearance shocked her family at a visit about a week before her death. It prompted her sister to return and stay overnight, so she was there with me at the moment of Irene's passing, holding Irene's other hand.

The doctor visited on Tuesday, May 29, Irene's fourth day in hospice care. He was a lighthearted sort, maybe intentionally, given his specialty. Irene was still able to kibitz a little with him. She was always ready to laugh or smile at someone's jokes. Later, when he was leaving, he pulled me aside and told me he did not think it would be three to six months. That was shocking to me. I prayed for much longer than the three to six months the oncologist anticipated. The hospice doctor said he would have a better estimate by the next time he came to the house, in four weeks or so. He didn't get to visit that second time. Irene passed away within three and a half weeks after the doctor's visit.

Irene worsened, as I explained. She only barely reached her arm over to touch me as we rested side by side in bed. She was unable to respond or help the nurse's aide in her own bathing by the third week.

Irene was silent most of the time, sleeping. As I was repeatedly told by the lead nurse, it was the natural process of dying. Irene did seem peaceful, hardly moving or speaking. The nurse told me at this time, June 20, that she did not believe Irene would manage to live another week. Nevertheless, she ordered the hospital bed the day before Irene died. She had to cancel the order. Less than forty-eight hours later, Irene breathed her last. And I, in a manner of speaking, died with her.

The Final Moments

I saw a decline in Irene's condition ever since we were told there was nothing else available for her treatment. Last year, we were told there would be no more surgeries. That was a dose of reality. Several surgeries had been available in the past. That notification was a milestone in our trek through the cancer treatment forest. But that latest message on May 25 was the worst.

I need to mention that Irene's reputation among my family members included her ability to find lost keys, eyeglasses, notebooks, and the like. She had an uncanny knack for knowing where the misplaced items could be located. Jewelry, scissors, refrigerator warranties, old photographs, Maria's old insurance policies, and other scattered documents never stayed lost for long. And Irene held on to what she considered her domain for as long as it was physically possible for her to search and do chores. But over the years, there was a slow transference of duties around the house, such as laundry, Dusty's litter box (he stayed with us to the end), vacuuming, and other household duties.

About a week and a half before she passed, Irene was able to get out of bed on two occasions: once when my sister and brother-in-law dropped by, and another time, when Irene's sister and brother-in-law visited. Irene would move heaven and earth to be out of bed when someone visited, despite how awful she felt. She was unable to get out of bed on the very last visits of each side of our families. A few in her family were shocked at how successfully Irene had hidden her suffering through the months they hadn't seen her. Irene always conversed by phone as if nothing was bothering her. She hid it well. On their final visits, they saw what they thought was a very sudden deterioration.

I observed Irene's physical and mental condition for years. I saw her in public, and I lived with her at home. I heard her scream in pain and then apologize for being so loud. I witnessed her being quiet for days, unable to gather the strength to get out of bed, and she apologized for that, too.

When at home, we used our solitude to comfort ourselves in our own nest and at appropriate times, we spoke of our wishes after our deaths. That subject is not a common one among folks, I understand, though it should be. It gave us a strange refuge from everything and everyone else. Others think about it but don't discuss it, for reasons that are built into our culture, I guess. Irene and I didn't dwell on the subject, but we confronted it.

What should I do with her Claddagh rings? What should the funeral be like, for either one of us, depending on who died first? Should it be burial or cremation? We made up our minds it should be cremation, and we confirmed it with her family also. Living wills, Do Not Resuscitate orders, last will and testament—what of those documents? Should there be a luncheon? Definitely not! Did everyone have the phone numbers of everyone else? What happens to all my books, hundreds of them that now can be completely contained in a couple DVDs with unused data storage left over. Volumes of books are a very heavy burden to relocate. They better stay *in situ*. How about the diamond in her engagement ring?

Irene wanted cremation, a priest and mass, and no fuss—that was all. She wanted no special attention. She did not want to be on display with viewers making the usual comments. "Doesn't she look great?" "They did a good job on her, didn't they?" You know the common remarks people make at viewings. We have all made those remarks or thought them.

Irene was the only one who was allowed to put makeup on Irene, certainly not a funeral director or embalmer. She did not want to be the center of attraction at either the funeral home or in the center aisle at the front of the church with the coffin lid open wide. No, that was not for Irene—or for me.

Irene and I discussed cremation a few times and what should happen to our ashes. Here is the plan we both liked and decided on. After we both died, our ashes would be mixed, holding out a small amount of her ashes to be given to Irene's sister, to be her family's caretaker. That was done later, at Irene's funeral. When I pass, each of my sons will receive a small urn. Then the rest of my ashes will be comingled with Irene's.

My family still owns one burial plot in a cemetery just outside Philadelphia. My parents and grandparents rest in that area. I've read that most cemeteries allow up to three or four urns in a single burial plot. It is my wish that Irene and I finally will rest with my family. My parents would have loved Irene but never met her. I'll introduce her to them, finally. But again, maybe they've met already.

Another of our objections to burial revolved around both of us seeing a lot of dead and decaying bodies through our years on the police force. It's not at all pretty. The thought of the "worms crawling in and the worms crawling out" versus cremation was a clincher for us, and it did not contradict the church. As long as a Catholic does not prefer cremation because of a *disbelief* in the resurrection of the body, he or she is not out of compliance with canon law.

We believed that the decaying process interrupted rather than supported the resurrection of the body. We believed it was the soul that lived on in spirit—I could tell a few stories of Irene's "presence." We reasoned that the body, even though it was a "temple" to receive sacraments through, goes to "dust" quicker without going through any corruptive putrefying process.

If the church still held to the belief that cremation interfered with God's ability to resurrect the bodies of the dead, I believe it sold God short for centuries. The church no longer clings to that belief, though. The church still holds loosely enforced regulations, not canon law, that the mass can't be a true high requiem mass if the ashes are present in the church. The mass has to be a "normal" mass, except under certain conditions. That was our situation. We had a normal mass. Irene did not care about the finer points between the different celebrations. She wanted a mass, and I arranged it. I think the only outward difference between the two masses is the color of the vestments worn by the priest and the use of incense.

Irene's family is Ukrainian Catholic, which has a connection to Rome and the Roman Catholic Church, not Eastern Orthodox. The Catholic pope in Rome is their highest prelate. When we were younger, the Catholic Church discouraged cremation. Since the 1960s there has been a relaxed attitude toward cremation and in 1997, I believe, it was deemed acceptable under certain conditions. There's plenty of information regarding every aspect of the entire process, practiced for more than twenty thousand years, including applicable canon and civil law.

Irene preferred cremation because of her reluctance to be center stage. Members of my eighth-grade class contacted me around December 2011, most of them for the first time in sixty years. Certain members of the class had decided to organize a sixtieth reunion. They found me and Irene and learned of our situation. The founding committee was starting a newsletter. Very sympathetically, the committee wanted to feature Irene and me in the very first issue. Irene declined the honor, saying that the first issue should be on a very positive note, not a sad one. "Maybe later," she said. That's the way she was. She did not need the limelight in any way, except with those she loved.

Irene did not want a luncheon after her funeral either, partially for the same reasons she preferred cremation. She believed that luncheon traditions often diminish some of the solemnity of the occasion. She'd attended a few luncheons when the memory of the deceased was not uppermost in the guests' minds. Old rivalries can surface. They can get out of hand easily. She also prayed that her family would get along. Her mother's care was constantly on her mind.

Irene became a spiritual person—not that she wasn't always a believer, but her spirituality became more overt. When her mother lived with us, we attended mass at St. Thomas Aquinas parish fairly regularly. For all the years after Irene was diagnosed, she prayed her novenas and rosaries. That provided her some inner comfort and contentment. I avoided interrupting her prayers as we drove to make an appointment for chemo or surgery. I considered Irene's praying a very personal time for her.

Our later drives were usually quiet and solemn. The same was true for our trips to her family in Bradenton. Even as she reclined the seat and curled up, she held rosary beads in her hands. "Prayer can't hurt," she would say. She looked like the angel she was, as I took my eyes off the road briefly to catch a glimpse of the woman I loved.

During the last night of her life, Irene lightly touched me with her left hand. In a very weak voice that pained me to hear, she said, "Tom"—that was all. At first, I interpreted it as Irene's needing help to get to the bedside commode. That was the first time that night Irene lifted and moved her arm over toward me. It was about 3:00 AM. I got up and went around to her side of the bed and put my arms around her to lift her. She uttered what I thought was, "No." I lay her back down and went to my side of the bed. I did not envision it might be close to the end. I was still expecting months—or weeks, at least.

A couple hours later, she reached her left arm over to me once again. This time her arm movement had very little strength to it. Her eyes were closed. Again, Irene simply said, "Tom."

I got up and went to her side and sat on the edge of the bed. She was very quiet and still. I watched her soft face with her lips parted slightly. I watched for yet another half hour.

You're so beautiful, honey. Please don't leave me.

"I love you, honey," I said aloud. "I love you, sugar."

After I told her I loved her, I quietly went back to my side of our bed.

As I write this, I admit my lips are quivering. Today, while thinking about that final night months ago, I wonder if it might have been her last plea. Was Irene letting me know she felt her death approaching? Maybe she wanted to tell me everything was fine and her pain was, at last, over after years and years of struggling. Maybe she wanted to assure me that she was okay and that I shouldn't worry. What was she trying to say? Lord, can I have those moments back please, just for a little while?

At 6:00 AM, I heard Irene's voice for the very last time.

"Tom."

I don't know what Irene's first words were as she made her way into this world and her troubled life. Maybe they were in Ukrainian; I don't know. But I do know the very last word Irene ever uttered in this world.

"Tom."

I got up again and went to her side of the bed. As I reached for her, I heard her deep breathing. Full of fear, I yelled for her sister to come downstairs. She had fortunately stayed overnight. Tammy hurried into the bedroom, and I told her to get on the other side of the king-sized bed and hold Irene's other hand—her left hand—and then lie down beside Irene.

I got a folding chair that I kept nearby for the hospice nurses during their exams and interviews with Irene. I sat beside the bed, on Irene's side, and phoned hospice. The representative told me to give her a particular pain medication. I put it into Irene's mouth and then got a can of Gatorade with a straw that I kept for her on the night table. I could see Irene make an effort to draw the soda up the transparent straw. It was a very weak effort, and she could bring the fluid only part of the way toward her pale lips.

Abandoning the suggestion, I took the pill from her mouth through her partially opened teeth. I had to use the end of a handy spoon. Her teeth were barely parted, too closed for me to reach my finger in to retrieve the pill. Irene's breathing continued with that raspy, tortured sound. I called hospice again and told them to rush a nurse. Tammy and I waited, holding Irene's hands.

I spoke to Irene, telling her I loved her and pleading for her to stay with us. "Don't leave me," I told her. "I'll care for you another nine years. We can keep on going, doing the same thing. We'll apply for other clinical trials. Something else will be discovered, a new miracle drug."

Irene's breathing did not improve. I made certain she was getting oxygen through her nose by adjusting the lines around her ears snugly—hoping, praying.

On that final morning, I saw almost two hours of deep breaths and then, five seconds of her obviously final, even deeper breaths—five of them—and then, nothing. I never want to witness that again.

My first call to the Hospice of the Comforter at 6:00 AM, evidently might not have been interpreted as a “final moments” phone call. Maybe they were not expecting Irene to pass so soon either. I called hospice again, and through my tears, I told them Irene had passed away. They dispatched our lead nurse. Over the next few hours, I felt Irene’s hand losing warmth.

I knew what death looked like. I knew the signs. Irene left this life at 8:20 AM on Friday, June 22, 2012. Just twenty-eight days passed since we were told she had three to six months to live. The official time of death was 9:30 AM, when the lead nurse arrived and conducted the required pronouncement.

Irene was very definitely one of a kind. So many women and men today are imitating movie stars or TV personalities. They imagine themselves as someone else. That’s a pity. Irene was so natural.

The lead nurse contacted the funeral home I chose. The funeral director arrived about an hour and a half later, near 11:00 AM. I’d been holding Irene’s hand since six o’clock that morning. I wish I’d had the right words to say during those long hours. I hope I did. I wish someone from hospice had been there all during that time—the chaplain or nurse or doctor, directing and guiding me. I know that’s an unreasonable wish. But it would have been comforting. Maybe they would have made me more certain that I was saying the right words. I don’t know if I ever will know if it would have helped.

In between my own convulsive sobs, when the lead nurse arrived I told her I had sometimes witnessed dying moments when I was on the police force, especially when I was a homicide detective. I didn’t know I would be so shocked. Inside my own mind, I’d known for a very long time that Irene’s case was terminal. It didn’t matter. Her death floored me. I could not catch my own breath. I couldn’t believe it. I still can’t. Every time I look at the brass urn on our dresser I compulsively shake my head in denial. *No. Not yet, Irene. Come back, please.*

Only a few days before, in the early evening, Irene and I spoke as we were lying side by side. It was no different from countless other evenings, though her words came haltingly. I didn’t realize it was our last pillow talk. Irene mentioned the surgery I needed for *my* hand. She made me promise I would get it done when she passed. She mentioned *my* stomach problems. She hinted that I should sell both cars and get a newer one for *myself*. Still, Irene was concerned about *me*. We had those same conversations in the past. There was nothing out of the ordinary. But Irene knew. I was unsuspecting, not at all ready for what was to come only days later.

I knew she was very weak, but I wasn't expecting this—so soon! Hadn't the doctors at Moffitt told us three to six months? Sure, the hospice nurse and doctor said it wouldn't be three to six months—but this? This was too soon! I was not prepared.

I was sobbing heavily. The nurse, who regularly witnessed the reactions of loved ones, said it was always a shock to the survivors who loved the deepest, regardless of how long it was anticipated.

When the funeral director removed Irene's body from our bedroom, he left a silk rose in her place. It is still there. I am unable and unwilling to remove it. The holy card with her picture and Sonnet XXIX also remains in the same place. So are all her clothes and shoes and personal makeup cases and paraphernalia. I can't disturb any of it just yet. I will, in time, not now. I kissed her on her lips before she was taken from the bedroom to the waiting hearse. But time passes and action needs to be taken. What must I do now?

Come back, honey. Please come back to me. Tell me what to do. Tell me what you want me to do.

A couple months later, Hospice of the Comforter sent me a questionnaire to complete. They wanted to know if their service was what I expected. I gave them high marks.

Necessities of Life—and Death

For me, the time between Irene's passing and her mass was full of sobbing and weeping while trying to make arrangements. I had a very difficult time talking to anyone. Everyone wanted to extend condolences and tell me how wonderful Irene was. When I heard the compliments, I would sense her loss even more. I suppose that the obituary in the newspaper and the hubbub of activity over the last days and morning in our driveway informed our neighbors and friends of

Irene's passing. The neighbors already knew Irene was battling cancer and knew her condition was severe.

My sister and brother-in-law, along with their extended family, came to our house immediately. They were tremendously helpful in guiding me through the motions of ensuring people were notified. One son flew into town; the other drove seventeen hours straight through to be with me. They stayed a full week, until after the services. I was grateful.

Irene's sister communicated through her side of her family. I really don't remember very much from the day of Irene's passing. I know I had things to do. I don't remember doing them. As the weekend continued, I arranged Irene's cremation, signed several releases and other state-required forms, and tried to give relatives information that they were clamoring for, which I didn't have yet.

The funeral home had to get approval for cremation from the state. That took at least a few days. The pastor of the church was on vacation. Other priests had to be rounded up. Reservations at the church had to be made, depending on whether or not the ashes would be available at the same time the church was available. We might have to do the mass without the ashes if the state didn't approve the cremation in time.

I had to get a framed picture, a bouquet of preferably white flowers, select the style of urns and holy cards (Irene's police picture and Sonnet XXIX), and keep everyone informed as to whether or not the mass would be on this day or that day, depending on which day the church scheduled its weekly cleaning and if a priest and soloist would be available.

Irene's family was anxious regarding the timing of the mass. Irene's mom, Maria, was delicately told of Irene's death. Saturday, June 30, was the best day all around. People were off work. Northerners and others could book flights or have time to make the trip by car. The 7th Police District in Philly arranged for a representative to attend the mass. The ashes would be available by that time.

One big headache was handled exclusively by the funeral director's aides who came to the church services. The funeral home's price included church fees, altar boys' tips, priest's honorarium, and all other various and sundry fees one never thinks of in these situations. I wrote a check for one lump sum; at least, I think I did. I don't really remember. I didn't have to worry about any of that at church.

Irene's Funeral Mass

On Saturday, June 30, 2012, we all went to Irene's celebratory mass at 11:00 AM. Naturally, my family and I were at the church at least a half hour early. There was an anteroom where we greeted arriving friends, neighbors, and relatives after they signed the guestbook. A lot of tears were shed in that room.

The mass was held in the regular church. The funeral parlor aides ushered everyone to the pews. My sister and Irene's sister brought the gifts of wine and water crucibles to the altar. I was instructed to carry the urn to the altar and place it on a small table in front of the communion rail. I took my place in the very front pew, next to the table where Irene's ashes, picture, and bouquet rested.

My sons took seats directly behind me. Maria sat four seats away in the same pew. Before we sat down, I asked my sons to take an opportunity to give Maria a hug. They loved her stories. She fascinated them. They were able to do so. So did I. Because she was in the front pew, as I was, I simply exited my seat and took three steps to be in front of her. She hugged me back.

Maria looked tiny. Her oldest son, a big man, had his arm around her shoulders, hoping to give her some comfort. Her tears flowed down the craggy, worry-worn cheeks of that eighty-eight-year-old woman who had suffered and seen so much tragedy in her life. And now, her youngest had died—her baby, Irene. What else would that woman suffer in the remainder of her troubled life?

I knew I would be unable to give the eulogy, even though up to a couple of days before mass, I was preparing for it. But maybe there wouldn't be a eulogy. However, when my brother-in-law and my sister picked me up for church, Don told me that he would deliver it. He was a lifesaver. Someone who knew her very well would give the eulogy.

Don's Eulogy

I have taken a lot of literary license in order to present the gist of Don's eulogy so that you can understand his intentions.

Good morning, everyone. I'm Don. I'm married to Tommy's sister, Pat. We knew and loved Irene. So did our sons and daughters and their families for about the last dozen wonderful years—ever since Tommy introduced her to our family.

Through my tears, I could tell Don was just a little nervous. He later mentioned to me that his hand was shaking so much he had a tough time writing his name in the guestbook when we arrived at church with the family. Later, when I had the guestbook at home, I hardly recognized his signature. Only because it was right under my sister's name was I able to see it was his John Hancock.

We could see she was a keeper from the beginning. She was so generous and always joining in the fun and laughter at our family gatherings. She was very much a part of our family.

Don stressed the word "keeper." We all knew what he was saying and what he meant. I heard the word too. Don had written out a few thoughts before mass, when he knew I was in no condition to give the eulogy, and no one else stepped forward. At first, he fidgeted a bit with his notes as he stood behind the lectern. I was proud to be his brother-in-law. He has always been like blood to me.

Irene never held back or shied away in showing her affection and deep love for Tommy and the rest of us, too. We loved that about her openness. That's the way she was with everybody. She never was first in her own eyes with anyone. It was never all about her. She was just a great listener.

She simply loved Tommy, and he adored her. That was obvious to anyone who knew him before Irene came into his life. Her love would light him up, and that was easy to see when they were together. We all loved her for the delight and pleasure she brought to Tommy's world from the very beginning, and we all knew the timing couldn't have been better. Remember, he was single for twenty years before he married her. Everyone could see the feelings they had for each other, just by watching them when they were together. Luckily, they had some time when they were able to enjoy life and be worry-free for a few years before Irene was diagnosed with cancer.

Through my tears and sobs, I could tell Don was settling down and getting in stride. His many years of experience as a manager at General Electric surfaced.

Their troubles began in August 2003 and for the next nine years—through doctor's appointments, all the prescriptions she had to take, blood draws, diagnostic and staging scans, hours and hours of chemo sessions with the awful side effects, short procedures, major surgeries with all the hospital stays, both up north and in Florida, feeding tubes, visits to the ER, and countless other problems that we don't even know about—through all of that, they hoped and prayed. So did we.

I heard Don emphasize each and every hardship as he listed them, and I listened.

Over the years, we were at their home many times, and they were at ours. We often visited her in the hospital, too. We never saw Irene whine or complain. She was always smiling. But there were times we could see the toll her ordeal was taking on her—and Tommy—especially after the awful hours of chemo. There were tears when she was given good news and tears of disappointment, too, when they were told that the cancer was back in the lung or the liver or her stomach. We were all heartbroken when that would happen.

I believe Don was misting up a tiny bit, as were others in the gathering, but I'm not sure of that. His words guided my mind as it floated back through my years with Irene. I still did not believe she was gone. I was sitting right beside the table on which I'd placed a framed photo of Irene in her police shirt and tie, a vase with a bouquet of white lilies, and the bronze urn containing her ashes. But I still could not believe it.

I fixed my eyes on the cross adorning the urn. I thought of the cross Irene and I saw on our trips on Interstate 4. I heard Maria crying to my right. I was in the first pew on the aisle. She was three or four seats in from the aisle. I briefly got out of my seat and went over the few feet between us, leaned over the front rail, and hugged her. Don paused just a brief moment. He saw what I was doing. Maybe he took the interlude to anticipate his next remarks. My back was toward him so I didn't really notice. Then I returned to my seat. It was a relief just to embrace Irene's mother for a moment.

Don, by this time, didn't need his notes anymore. He was really delivering the eulogy with the memory of Irene, and the words and phrases came from his heart. I loved Don for more than fifty years as a member of our family. His genuine emotion was coming through to me and everyone else who was listening.

Don hurriedly picked his handkerchief from inside his jacket and dabbed his brow, I think. He then continued, still holding his hanky, while bracing the podium with his hands.

Irene and Tommy often told us they wanted quantity from the doctors, hoping for new cures. They would try to make their own quality. Tommy was there every step of the way—nine years of total caring.

Last year, for months and months, fifteen hours a day, Irene had to be hooked up to a feeding tube. We remember when the pump for the feeding tube would kink and jam, and the fluid wasn't going through. It would beep all day and night long. We were there. We heard it. Irene wasn't getting all the nutrition or rest she needed. They would have to get with the supplier and luckily, they finally replaced the pump. We were there when it was delivered.

In spite of all the hardship and pain, Irene kept her sense of humor. Now and then we would get a good laugh when she would lay on us a tale or an Irene-ism. Here are a few I remember:

Besides having to rush her to the ER several times, about a year ago, Tommy couldn't get Irene to respond when she was in the bathroom. Tommy had to dial 911, unlock the front door, and then quickly get back to Irene. He was trying to get her back on the bed. He managed to get her partway on the bed when he could tell she was beginning to come around. Just then, he heard the EMTs coming into the house. He yelled and told them where Irene was. Four big men, fully equipped, came into their bedroom. Tommy told them about the situation.

One of the team started asking the normal questions: "What's your name?" Irene mumbled. "What's today's date?" Irene mumbled. "What day of the week is it?" "I don't know," Irene said. "Maybe Tuesday?" "Who's the president of the United States?" one of the firemen asked. "Ohhhh! Please! Don't make me feel any sicker than I already am." She blurted those words out with her usual smile. The fireman laughed and took her vital signs. They said they didn't think she needed to go to the ER. She was alert again.

Don made me reflect on why it was so easy for me to be around Irene. Like me, Irene was fiscally conservative. That should be no surprise, given her background. She had to watch her bankbook very carefully most of her life. That made life so much easier between us. Being debt-free is true freedom. It sure is a plus if both people have the same ideas about money. I recommend partners be on the same page, not only fiscally but politically as well. It's great if they share most other belief systems, too, especially values.

I'll mention another time we got a look into Irene's humor. I'm a Disney van driver, part-time. I've been chauffeuring visitors around the Disney property for ten years. I know all the shortcuts to wherever the visitors want to go. At one of our family gatherings, I was wondering when I should retire and when I would know the right time. You know, we cast members get free passes that we can use to get family and friends into the parks. It's been a great benefit over the years for us. That's tough to give up. Well, when Irene and the rest of us were sitting around the table on the lanai, Irene answered my question: "You'll know when you ask the passengers where they want to go and when they tell you to take them to Magic Kingdom, you ask them how to get there!" Our family crowd cracked up.

Over those nine years, Irene and Tommy made the best of a bad situation. Irene's strength was amazing. They went to the California wine country twice, to Vegas, all over Florida, back and forth and in between up north and Florida, and even to Ireland. They used to say the Ukraine was next.

As time went by, Irene had a tough time flying—or even on long drives. Eventually, over the last couple years, she had to tote along a bedside basin whenever she even went on the one-and-a-half-hour drive to the cancer hospital for appointments. She still did all that suffering in silence. And she was always thinking of others, even animals. There was Dusty. Irene worried about who would take care of her mother, Tommy, and of course, her cat. She loved Dusty. She knew Tommy would be going up north a lot on extended stays to visit his sons, afterward. Irene knew that. Her sister promised to take care of Dusty. Irene really reminded me a lot of Tommy and Patsy's mother, my mother-in-law, during the last months of each of their lives—quiet suffering, never complaining ... except about the hospital food.

Even the hospice lead nurse admitted to me and Patsy that at first, she did not believe it when we told her about all the surgeries Irene had. Then she saw all the scars. She said the tumors were so big that they bulged out from Irene's stomach. Tommy told us that over the last several months, Irene told him that she knew how bad things were for her when she could feel and see the size of the tumors on her liver.

There's no way I can end without mentioning a couple other traits Irene had. She loved to please others. It showed in her cooking when, early on, she hosted get-togethers at their home. She missed being able to do that as time went on. And what a work ethic: power-washing, cleaning the bird poo off the pool screen, potting and repotting plants on the lanai, and don't stand still too long, or you might get painted along with the lanai and the house. Irene never put any dishes in the dishwasher unless she'd already washed and sanitized them. She always wanted to help whenever she came to our home, too, no matter how bad she felt. She wouldn't let anyone know how she was feeling, and she would just jump in to help. She was simply one of a kind.

Irene could also listen to Tommy's commenting on the politics of the day and, at the same time, make note of all the ingredients in a recipe on the Cooking Channel.

To let you know how much Irene was loved by everyone in our family, Tommy and Patsy's brother, Michael, has turned to writing books since he retired from the police force. In his last book, which will be published soon, he paid tribute to Irene. He knew how much disappointment she felt when she had to take herself off the promotion list. He created a character named Detective Irene Stasurak. Stasurak was her maiden name, you all know. Michael meant it to be a surprise for Irene. But Irene passed away before she was able to see herself as a detective. She wanted that gold shield. My brother-in-law Mike gave it to her.

Finally, I'll end with this:

Don paused for a moment as he collected his thoughts and then continued, full of emotion. He was talking to Irene.

You know, Irene, your Tommy always joked that he married you because of your foreign accent.

Don continued in character—he tried to imitate Irene's Philly twang.

And by the way, Irene, How ya doin'? We all hope you're finally out of pain and at peace. You deserve a break from what you've been through. We all wish we could have another cup of "cawfee" with you, too, at least one more cup.

Irene, thanks for the memories and for coming into our lives and giving us the wonderful pleasure of your company. We cherished every minute. We all miss you dearly, and all of us will love you forever.

Don slowly left the podium. He was a little emotional, I believe, over those last several sentences he addressed to Irene, but he managed to vocalize them. I'm not sure if anyone else had a dry eye; I certainly didn't. I could only see the little table with Irene's picture and the brass urn on the table's surface. It was in front of me and slightly to my left side. I couldn't take my eyes away. Finally, I looked at Don again as he took his seat.

Everyone at mass could appreciate his feelings toward Irene. I was extremely grateful to Don for giving the eulogy. I was completely unable to do it, even though I thought I could at fleeting moments during the week between Irene's death and the solemn mass. There was really no way. I was out of it.

Don's moving tribute to Irene was one of the most wrenching segments to relate in this book. I recalled his state and my own as he spoke, and I listened in those somber surroundings. I relived the moment. There were other chapters, of course, and sub-chapters that tore at me emotionally as I wrote. But overall, I believe that remembering my life with Irene and writing about it has been valuable therapy for my grief. Writing takes time and focus. And Irene will live on in my mind, heart, and soul forever. She will live on in these words also. This book will never go out of print. That is the publisher's business practice and promise.

The Continuing Presence of Irene

It's a common belief in some of the religions of the world that the soul of a loved one lives on in an afterlife. According to that system, in situations of the deepest love, "crossing over" becomes possible. It's always a choice whether or not to embrace that conviction. It's up to each individual. It can't be proven or disproven.

I recently took a trip up north to meet with relatives and friends who had sent their condolences but were unable to attend Irene's funeral mass. I flew up there and stayed with my son and his beautiful wife for eight days. I wanted to touch base with friends and relatives and thank them for any gifts they made in Irene's name to the hospitals and cancer institutes, which I had requested in lieu of flowers. That was Irene's wish, too. Irene always encouraged me to take the trip to see my boys. She suggested I take my son to Ireland, remember, when she couldn't make the trip herself a second time.

On the list to visit was Irene's friend and coworker, Sandy. She was the one who rescued the Ukrainian eggs when Irene was leaving her first husband—and most notably, the friend who had "hooked up" Irene and me in Atlantic City on one of the best days of my life.

Sandy and I decided to meet for lunch at a diner on Frankford Avenue. There's a driveway into which traffic turns from the avenue to get into the shopping center and then into the diner's parking lot. The driveway runs about fifty yards before a customer can make a right-hand turn into the restaurant's private lot. I was waiting along that stretch of the driveway. At first, I didn't recognize a car that had its passenger window rolled down. Then I heard the driver yelling for me to "get in, get in!" Of course, it was Sandy. I got into her car. There was still a little way to drive before she could park in the lot.

She was shouting, "I'm freaking out. This is too weird. Listen to the radio. I'm freaking out!"

There was a song that included in the lyrics the name Irene. As she continued toward a parking space, she said that she listened to that music station every day and hadn't heard that song in ten years. "I'm freaking out. I'm freaking out!" she kept screaming. I got chills. She said the song came on the moment she spotted me waiting as she turned into the driveway from the avenue.

"Irene is with us. She wants to have lunch with us like before. She wants to join us. Tom, I really, really miss her."

That lunch was dramatic. I told her a couple other stories in which I'd felt Irene's presence. I mentioned the heron wars. She remembered Irene's constant annoyance about that bird. When they would talk on the phone, now and then, Irene would interrupt their conversation to say that she or I needed a minute to chase the heron away.

This heron plagued Irene and me with his massive doo-doo deposits on our pool screen, some of which would leak onto the lava rock on the edging of the pool. The mess permanently stained the decorative stones. If I could ever hate one of God's creatures, it would be that bird. He had a long wart protruding from his throat, so he was easily recognizable and distinctive from the many other herons in the area. He was the only one who landed on our screen!

He usually sat on the edge of the screen, mostly at night. I saw him during the afternoon of the day that Irene died. He was turned toward the house a bit on his perch, as if he wanted to know what all that activity was on the lanai. Maybe he was wondering why neither Irene nor I was chasing him away, as usual. It was a game I believe the heron enjoyed.

After a few minutes, that big blue heron just flew away, looking back over his wing at my family and me, as we sat somberly on the lanai. Did he sense tragedy? Did he realize Irene had died? Would he miss her? Regardless, I have not seen him since. It has been more than seven months. All the other wildlife that constantly parades before us is still there. The scenery is a wonderful benefit of Florida living that Irene and I fully enjoyed—except for that heron.

Maybe the disappearance of that particular bird was Irene's first afterlife effort to rid me of the menace. Sandy stated that the episode sounded like something Irene would take on, now that she might be able to. "Irene is still looking after you, Tom, by doing you that favor," she said. She was tickled that Irene was continuing to take care of me and joining us for lunch. She loved the bird story. We both miss Irene a lot. I bought a butter cake at the diner's bakery and went off to my next promised visit.

Sandy would enjoy this next story, too, even though she is of a different faith than Irene and me. I haven't spoken to her since I was up north, so she'll have to wait until the next opportunity I have to travel.

We Catholics are fortunate. We have patron saints for guiding us in what some call our charming and quaint belief system. One of them, Saint Anthony, traditionally known all over the world as the patron saint for lost articles, has nothing over Irene. Let me illustrate. Keep in mind the sub-chapter, "Final Moments," where I describe Irene's knack for finding misplaced items.

Yesterday, I picked up my mail and returned to my man/woman cave in the third garage. We only have two cars, so the remaining area, naturally, became a man/woman cave for me and my golf buddies through the years, including our wives.

While sitting there, I read a card from one of my grandnieces and her boyfriend. The cover of the card read, "Just checking in …" On the inside of the card was the rest of the sentence: "to see how you're doing." And below, she had written: "Just a note to let you know we're still thinking about you." I once told this grandniece that she does some of the same things Irene used to do. The card was a gesture that Irene would have done in the same situation. Was Irene hinting? You tell me after you hear the story.

As I was sitting there reading the note, my sister called. She wanted to know if I wanted to go to a matinee to see a movie that just came out. Irene and I always preferred the afternoon matinees when we went to the movies. On top of that, this was a movie Irene and I had been waiting to see. It was Part II of *Atlas Shrugged*. Irene and I had seen Part I earlier in the year. Pat said that I would have to leave right away to meet her and Don at the theater in time.

No problem. I dropped everything and drove to the shopping center where the movie house was located. They paid the steep price but got a Disney employee discount, and I didn't object. Don and Pat led the way to seating, not me. We bypassed the popcorn stand. Don took us to the last row and sat in the same seats where Irene and I always sat. In this particular theater, there was more leg room, and it was more comfortable for Irene. And the last row was always available at matinees. While sitting there, I was going to dutifully turn off my cell phone, but I noticed I had a message from my sister, who was sitting immediately beside me. I hadn't looked at messages for a couple days. But I looked on this occasion.

I nudged Pat showing her the e-mail on my cell phone screen. She said she'd forwarded those e-mails to me a couple days ago. She received them, at that time, from each of my two grandnieces, Jenny and Meghan—"g-nieces" for short. Pat, who was g-mom to my g-nieces, told me to read them in a certain sequence. I began to read the first e-mail that I hadn't opened in the intervening days. Jenny wrote:

"So, I have been watching a lot of [the TV show] *Long Island Medium*, and she says those who have crossed over will make it known if they are around you. Well, I was cleaning my room, and I was cleaning my chest of drawers out. Something fell when I pulled the drawer open, and it was a birthday card from Uncle Tommy and Irene. What's strange is, I rarely keep birthday cards. That's not the best part. Two days later, guess what I found—my diamond earring! It was the one I lost like six months ago, the pair of silver hoops with the diamonds in them that you, g-mom, and g-pop gave me for Christmas. I couldn't believe it. I have been carrying the one earring in my wallet since the day I lost the other one. Then right after I found it, I turned around and opened my end table to clean it out. Guess what was there—Irene's mass card. I think it was Irene who found the earring."

Pat heard my soft sobs. I don't think anyone else did. The theater was not crowded at all. I don't think Don heard them either from two seats away. They were more like quiet whimpers.

Irene, the finder of lost articles, was at it again, if one chooses to believe it. My family and I have all made that choice on several occasions. Pat whispered to me to read the other, shorter e-mail from my other g-niece—the one who sent me the card "checking in" by snail mail that I had just read an hour previously. She was adding on to her sister's e-mail, describing Irene's help in finding the earring.

Here it is:

"And to add to that, I just happened to mail Uncle Tommy a card yesterday to see how he's doing. This is all Irene's doing."

If I put it all together, what do I get? I have the "Just checking in ..." card from one g-niece, dated two days before I read it. That was Irene coaching my g-niece to see how I'm doing, using one of Irene's usual, thoughtful gestures. Then, at the same time I was reading and thinking about that nice card, my sister called to check if I wanted to go to the movies to see a show she knew Irene and I wanted to see and that we had previewed for Pat and Don. That was Irene telling Pat and Don to check on me and get me out of the house to see that movie. That's Irene still looking after her hubby, no doubt.

Irene always did worry about me. She worried about my health and well-being during her life and now, maybe afterward? I've mentioned her two greatest concerns did not include her own illness; she worried that she would not live long enough to take care of her mother, Maria, and me. That was the way she was, the most unselfish woman in the world.

I was sitting beside my sister in those special seats, when I obediently shut down my cell phone when prompted to do so on-screen. My sister forwarded two older messages from my g-nieces, but I hadn't read them until the moment I was sitting beside my sister. We were in seats Irene and I always chose when we would go to the movies. Further, at the exact moment I closed down my phone, I saw the messages. Normally in the movies, I would just shut it off without looking for any communications. In addition, my sister told me to read them before I turned off my phone because they were important.

You can decide if Irene is still around. I think the messages speak for themselves. Do you think Irene was there with us, watching Part II? She really wanted to see it. She was a persistent type, you know. When Irene wanted to or needed to, she could be very determined. She had a very strong personality. Do you think the deep love we all had for each other enabled her to cross over? I guess we'll see, as time goes on.

I love believing in these associations, as did Irene when she was alive. It's not healthy to have *too* much logic guiding you through life's tributaries. You have to have a nice blend of body, heart, mind, and soul. Maybe it's all part of our healing.

In one sense, it was so wonderful to be around Irene while she was intensely absorbing her last sights, sounds, and feelings on this earth. She knew she was dying. She wanted to internalize and have it all sink into her very bones. Irene, when she could, enjoyed everything as if it were the first time she was experiencing the world around her. Few can truly empathize with how she viewed her world since she was told she had only three to six months to live. Most can't put themselves into Irene's shoes. They don't think about dying. If you know how to die, I guess you can figure out how to live.

Fortunately, my family reached out to Irene and me during the past nine years. We always tried to have fun together. Topics of discussion were lighthearted and usually funny—a typical Irish reaction to the world around us. Word games and trivia, along with a few beers and wine, were enough to keep Irene and me smiling and laughing when we visited my family. As you can see, my family continues to be at my side. We find Irene's presence around us all the time. She will always be with us—and me.

What? Hello … hello … hello. Honey, was that you? Where are you?

Ah! There you are. I knew you'd show up. I just knew it!

"Hi, honey."

Hi, handsome.

Postscript

Conversations

I'm having a nice conversation with Irene. She has some questions for me, and I have many for her. Irene is interested in several areas:

1. Her mother, Maria: how is she doing? Her mom's well-being and care were always a grave concern of hers. Has her mom adjusted? How about everyone else in Bradenton? And Dusty, of course.
2. My health: am I okay? Have I adjusted? Am I taking my meds for high blood pressure and diabetes regularly? Irene always ensured I followed the orders. Did I get my hand surgery? What about that ablation procedure for my esophagus? Is my stomach doing better? Irene is reminding me to schedule my next colonoscopy soon and to tell Tommy and Chris not to wait too long before they schedule their own colonoscopies. It's in the family. She is telling me to fly up to see the boys real soon.
3. Did I give her Claddagh rings to her sister and my sister? What did I do with her engagement ring diamond? Did I have it mounted in a new college ring, like she suggested?

"But honey, I'd like to know about your final moments. Irene, it happened too suddenly. We weren't able to have a final, complete conversation. I wanted to tell you more. I wanted to know your thoughts. Were you comfortable and peaceful? What was it like? Could you hear me telling you I loved you? Could you feel me holding your hand? Did you know Tammy was with us?"

Irene is telling me she will answer my questions after I answer hers, all in good time. She said she doesn't have a lot of time on this visit. She thinks she will be called soon. Did you hear her?

She knows I feel her presence all the time. She is aware that my family, now and then, senses her but isn't certain if she has gotten through.

"The girls know it was you who helped in finding that earring, honey."

I tried to cross over a couple times. I wasn't sure ...

"You got through, honey! And thank you for getting the heron to fly away and never come back. That's one mess I don't have to deal with anymore. And yes, honey, your mom is doing well. I swear she will outlive all of us. She can still jump fences. She had her eighty-ninth birthday a month ago. She misses her baby, but I took the notice that the funeral home created with your picture on it and put it in a nice frame. That announcement is the last picture in the photo section that I included in your book. When I gave it to her, here in our family room, she clutched it to her heart and wept a bit. Then she turned to me and wanted to make sure I had a duplicate of my own. I showed her my copy hanging on the wall in the hall. She smiled. I want you to know she is fine, hon. Please, don't worry.

"Then I took your mom into our bedroom and showed her your urn. She caressed it and touched the cross mounted on the front of it. I showed her the silk rose I keep on your side of the bed. She gently held it in her small hand and laid it back in the same position. She was strong, but she couldn't keep a tear or two from trickling out of her misty eyes onto her cheeks. She put her fingertips on your police badge that I leave beside the urn. Then we went back to the family room where your nephew and his wife were waiting to take her back to Bradenton. That was very nice of them to bring her over here.

"Dusty is holding his own over there, too, beautiful. Don't worry about him."

And you, Tommy?

"Me, honey? I'm doing fine. Writing this book has been very pleasant therapy and occupied me intensely at times. It's been almost seven months. Of course, I have my moments when I fill up. The first time was a few days after everyone learned of your passing, Mike called me and told me he had wanted to surprise you with the creation of a new female character in his latest novel, *Imperfect Contrition*. He named her Detective Irene Stasurak. That was such a touching gesture. Mike wished the book had been published in time for you to be surprised and to flash your usual broad and happy smile a little broader at finally getting your gold badge, at least vicariously."

Please thank him for me, Tom—sincerely. That was so nice. He didn't have to do that. I'll have to ask everyone up here to call me detective from now on.

"Up here?"

I'll talk to you privately about that a little bit later. It's very, very personal, as it should be—with the readers, too.

"Another time, a month after you passed, we went up to Maureen's. By the way, her son, Sean, told me he misses playing cards with you. He just turned eleven a couple months ago. Maureen told me that she got involved with the Relay for Life for the American Cancer Society up in Mount Dora, Florida, on April 20, 2013. So I quietly said that was nice. I think I was in another zone. Then she added she would be a team leader of about five groups. Again, in that same zone, I said that was nice. Finally, she told me the name of her team was Team Irene. Well, I had to go out to the patio when she told me that. I filled up. Pat also couldn't hold back the tears, great comforting sister that she is.

"That was such a great tribute to you, honey. Maureen also created a link at American Cancer Society's webpage for people to participate and donate. I'm going to bring copies of your book to give away and sign. I hope it is published and available by that deadline.

"Later that evening, Maureen apologized because she hadn't considered how recent your death had been. I told her that was not the cause of my composure failing a bit. It was the impact I felt that others in my family were also feeling your loss, honey. I wasn't alone. They all loved you so much.

"Several times while writing the book, it was kind of rough. But I am adjusting. I still miss you, as I always will. You brought into my life an experience few have. You showed me how to love, which was only a dream before you came into my life. What a great gift that was, Irene.

Thank you for that privilege. And even now, you are why I can believe in angels, sugar.

“Yes, I’m taking my meds pretty close to on time every day. I have an appointment next month for that diabetes check-up—the A1C blood glucose. The ablation of my esophagus, the third and last one, went well. That was less than a month ago. Pat took me to and picked me up from the hospital—like you did on the last day you ever drove. Thank you, Irene, for doing that for me, despite how bad you were feeling. I think you knew that it might be the last act you could do for me. Thank you, honey.

“The boys have come down twice since June, once for your funeral when they stayed for a week; and once to just visit and keep me company. They were making certain I was doing okay. I’ve been up North twice. The first time, I wanted to see those friends and relatives who could not make it down for your funeral. I wanted to personally thank everyone for the donations they made to cancer organizations and hospitals in your name, as I requested. I went to my sixtieth grade school reunion, too. All my classmates offered their sympathy, honey. I appreciated it. Then, the second time was just to visit Tommy and Christopher. They are both doing very well.

“Oh! I had lunch with our matchmaker, Sandy, who felt your presence while I was with her. I’ll have to remember to tell you about that before you have to go. Let me get back to Tommy and Chris just now.

“Chris landed his first full-time RN job as a supervisor—big bucks! Tommy is a regional manager with a large company—big bucks! I told them I wouldn’t be up there again until the weather is a lot warmer. I froze on my last trip in late November and early December. I reminded them about getting colonoscopies no later than age forty. Colon cancer is in the family. They miss you. Tommy’s Irene and her parents also miss you. Everybody misses you, honey. Everybody loves you.”

The rings and my diamond, Tom?

“Yes, Irene, here’s what I did with the Claddagh rings and your diamond. First let me show the ring to you.”

It’s so beautiful, Tom. I love what you did with it. It captures our friendship, our careers, our engagement, our marriage, and our life together. I love it.

"Now I'll show you the original sub-chapter I wrote, intending to include it somewhere in the book. I thought the readers would enjoy it. It expresses the love in our relationship so beautifully. But I didn't feel as though it fit anywhere in the book. I just couldn't find the right place. Now that you asked, though, I think I'll just read it to you, and at the same time, I'll be letting the readers know what happened. Tell me if you like it, honey. I'll read it now. Are you sure you have time, honey?"

Yes, Tom. Please read to me like you used to.

"Okay. Here it is, as it would appear in your book.

The Claddagh Rings and the Diamond

"Claddagh is a small fishing village just outside Galway on the west coast of Ireland. Irene and I were there. The village claims to be the place where the Irish Claddagh design originated. A Google search will fully explain the long tradition of the famous rings. But now, I want to focus on why our rings were important to Irene and me.

"First, let me describe the classic yet modern Claddagh ring. Traditionally, it is gold, not any other metal, if it is given as a significant symbol to a loved one. Three major components compose the design: a heart, symbolizing love; a crown above the heart, denoting loyalty; and a pair of hands on either side of the heart, cradling it. The hands tell of friendship and have frilly cuffs at their wrists. The two sides are connected with the band surrounding the finger.

"In Ireland, unmarried and available individuals wear the ring on their right hand, with the heart's lower point facing toward the fingertips, denoting the wearer is very available, or with the heart pointing toward the wrist, sending a message that the wearer is probably taken. In the United States, as in Ireland, the rings are usually worn as friendship, engagement, or wedding rings on the left ring finger. If the crown is toward the wrist on the left ring finger, that can mean the wearer is engaged or taken—not married.

"If the crown is toward the fingertips and the heart, therefore, is toward the wrist—that is, the wearer's heart—it usually signifies it is a wedding band or the wearer is committed. There are exceptions to the above practices, of course. Some people simply like the ring's intrinsic beauty and symbolism. They wear them as they choose, disregarding any personal intent.

"I've mentioned the Claddagh rings that Irene and I both wore, denoting our relationship to each other. The rings are important to those of Irish heritage, though other ethnic groups also appreciate what the rings symbolize. Irene, for example, though Ukrainian, treasured the two gold Claddagh rings I gave her. One was a friendship ring, the other an engagement ring. The latter, after marriage, became a wedding band when Irene turned the heart's point toward her own heart. The ring can play a dual role, depending on whether the point of the heart is toward the wrist or fingertips and which hand it is worn on."

I loved it when you first gave me that friendship ring. I felt young and pretty.

"You're getting ahead of the story, honey. I'll continue.

"Irene and I both wore our rings as wedding bands after we were married. Initially, I gave Irene a plain gold Claddagh as a friendship ring. I know, that's old-fashioned, but so were we. Then I gave her a fancier one. The heart was filled with little sparkling chips. It was very pretty. And following tradition, I also gave her a normal engagement ring with a diamond, just about a carat."

Tom, excuse me, but you don't know how much that lit up my life when you gave me that friendship ring. It made me feel like a teenager again. We were old-fashioned, weren't we? I loved that feeling. But Tom, I interrupted you again. Please, go on.

"Do you like it so far, honey?"

Yes, I do—very much so.

"Okay. I'll continue again.

"After we were married, Irene wore the traditional engagement ring with the bigger diamond when we dined out or at other social affairs. But on an everyday basis, she wore the Claddagh with the little chips on her left hand, with the heart pointing toward her heart. For our wedding, Irene gave me a Claddagh with a diamond, about .30 carat in the heart, set with a bezel. I wore it on my left hand, heart toward my heart.

"What should I do with Irene's Claddagh rings? Irene decided that question before she passed away. The engagement ring, the one with the chips, will go to my sister to match an earring and necklace set she owned. The friendship ring will go to Irene's sister. Now, what should I do with Irene's diamond ring?

"The diamond is about a carat. It shouldn't go to waste and sit in a drawer. Irene, thinking ahead, in spite of my refusal to do so (I hope you can understand my refusal), came up with an idea: replace my lost college ring, and then have the diamond set in the middle of that ring's stone.

"I liked that idea. I always wanted to get another college ring. It took me more than ten years to earn the first one. I lost it way back in the '70s. Today, its value is probably twenty times what I paid for it.

"I needed to find a jewelry store. Irene and I love this little town a few miles down the road from our home. Downtown St. Cloud has its antique shops; a special coffee and tea restaurant, whose owners want the sitting area to be considered a customer's second living room; a few other special, friendly, family restaurants on Pennsylvania Avenue, New York Avenue, and 13th Street; and a quaint English-style tearoom that also sells crafts and antiques, all owned by locals. And it seems like there's a barber shop for every other person. There are so many of them!

"The movie theater is classic. It's only open on weekends during the school year. Far from plush seating, Irene and I still sometimes preferred it over the glitzy theaters at Disney and elsewhere. You might expect to see a film from the silent-movie era playing there or *The Perils of Pauline*, but the movies are always some of the latest first-runs.

"There is even a marina and a two-block-long beach on the St. Cloud side of the lake. The sand spreads along the southern end of a circular lake that is about nineteen miles in circumference. We took Irene's mother, Maria, on an airboat ride on the lake. She loved it and saw a few alligators during that jaunt. There is a two-mile–long bike and jogging path, too. I walk it, of course."

I used to wait for you on a bench, Tom. I fed the ducks while I waited. Remember?

"Yes, honey, I do. I wish you were still on the bench with me. …

"A few weeks after Irene's funeral mass, I went online to see if I could get my college ring. It was too much trouble. I had an idea. In my searching, I saw a site on which I could design a law enforcement ring. I could select from scales of justice and other symbols for the side panels and have "Philadelphia Police" surrounding the stone of my choice. I ordered one. It took six weeks, and when it arrived, it was inscribed with my name. I thought it was just what I wanted. Maybe the jeweler could mount the diamond in the stone. Irene and I were both law enforcement. With her diamond in my ring, we would be joined again. I was on a quest.

"Be patient, honey. There's a little diversion here in the story for a minute.

"The diamond was too big for the small flat surface of the multifaceted synthetic stone. However, all was not lost.

"The jeweler's assistants joined in my quest. I had initially visited this jeweler because I had confidence in his shop and his helpers.

"I had confidence because of the way they took care of Irene's bracelet. I had given Irene a scarab bracelet—the scarab had belonged to my mother—but Irene lost one of the scarabs. Before she passed, Irene told me, with a wry smile, to have it repaired and then give it to Pat after the 'dust' settled—always a bit of humor.

"A week or so later, the assistant called and said the bracelet was ready. She had a rock, a lapis lazuli, from which she cut the stone to size and then sculpted the image of the beetle onto its surface. What a great job.

"That's not all. When I gave the bracelet to my sister, I told her the story. She asked if I thought the jewelry shop could convert an old set of earrings from the screw-on type to the pierced type. The earrings and necklace were heart-shaped with little diamond chips in the hearts. The set resembles closely the Claddagh ring with the chips that Irene wanted Pat to have. But she couldn't wear the earrings; they hurt.

"I took them to the shop in St. Cloud. Again, a week or so later, the job was done with anti-infection stainless-steel posts at a very modest price. Pat was very happy. She can now wear the fifty-year-old set, and Don can finally admire the entire gift he bought for her so long ago—and it is a match with her new Claddagh ring that Irene wanted her to have. Pat wears Irene's ring every day now.

"The assistants and owner knew that Irene had passed away and liked the idea of the sentimental memento I was trying to create. This time a third assistant attended to me. I could tell from her expression that she liked my story. She knew I was grasping for a solution.

"Through her constant smile, she offered an idea: how about if they took my Claddagh wedding band and its little .30 carat diamond and mount it on a more mannish ring (that is, a bigger one), so that it would be large enough to house my entire Claddagh. She diligently searched through her catalog books and found the perfect choice. It was a man's gold ring, with the face shaped like a police shield or badge. She knew of our law enforcement background.

"She said the designer could take Irene's one-carat diamond, place it in my Claddagh's heart, and put my little diamond at the point on the bottom of the shield. My Claddagh would be cut off at the cuffs and shaped to adhere to the flat, main surface of the new ring.

"I'm almost finished, honey.

"The man-sized ring was delivered in about a week, and I was summoned for an appearance. They were as eager as I was. They wanted to get started on it if I said to go ahead with it.

"The ring was a match. It would fit. I said to go ahead with the plan. Everyone agreed. A few weeks later, it was completed. I could not possibly be happier with the way it turned out. It was beautiful.

"Stay with me, Irene. Here comes the whipped cream and the cherry on the top. This will be a surprise for you."

I'm with you, Tom. Don't worry. What is the surprise?

"There was only one thing left to do. I wanted an inscription on the inside of the band: Irene's four-digit police badge number and to make it even more special, "I. C. ♥ T. C." to complete it."

Tom, that's beautiful. I wish I could kiss you. Thank you, handsome. We will be together, always. That ensures it!

"I'll continue, honey. There's just a little bit more.

"There it was, all in one beautiful setting—a police shield representing many years of our lives involved with law enforcement; my wedding Claddagh with a diamond that Irene gave me; her engagement diamond that I gave her; an inscription with her police badge number; and finally, our initials with a love/heart symbol between them. The sequence of the initials indicates that my Claddagh, the major component of the creation, was a gift to me from Irene. I couldn't wait to show my family.

"A couple days after I picked up my new ring, I was on a plane to Philly. Pat and Don took me to the airport. They were the first family members to see the ring. Their eyes lit up. They knew what the entire presentation meant to me.

"By the way, honey, all the Cooneys and Scullions up north were truly saddened by your passing. I could tell."

I always enjoyed their company, Tom. They are such nice people.

"I know. Okay, I'll continue now.

"Everywhere I went up North reminded me of places Irene and I had visited together in the past: Peddler's Village, New Hope, Newtown, Princeton, Bowman's Tower, and Washington's Crossing. She would have loved to visit the Amish market in Newtown that Tommy and I newly discovered. I also had a milkshake at Tanner's Market. A few years earlier, at Tanner's, Irene waited for me in the car. She wasn't feeling very well and was afraid of being sick inside the crowded store. I went inside to get some of that fabulous homemade ice cream. Memories—they were all around me."

I remember that, Tom. Yes. I wasn't feeling too good. I was a little afraid of upsetting the shoppers if I had to get sick inside. That would have been quite a scene. Then, you know me, I'd have to clean up my own mess. You parked near a little grass plot. That was a good location, just in case. I'm sorry again, handsome, for interrupting. Finish telling about the rings and diamond.

"Everyone up North who saw the design and heard the story was absolutely fascinated. When I returned to Florida, I just had to go to the jewelry store on New York Avenue to tell them how much everyone loved their work. The jewelry team deserves the accolades my family members gave them. I could tell they put their hearts into it. So did the artist. He had to make it all come together."

Tom, tell the people in the jewelry store how much I love the ring. Tell them thank you for me, please.

"I will, honey. Well, that's it. You're always such a polite listener, honey. Thank you. Well, what do you think?"

Irene is nodding, with a beautiful, proud smile on her face. She tells me to be sure to add it to the book, because it tells something more, something deeper, about our relationship and our love.

"Good! I'm glad you like it, beautiful."

Irene is now asking about my hand operation.

"Look at my hand, sugar. My fingers point straight up!"

That's terrific, sweetheart.

"And here, Irene, look at this. I wrote it for the book, but like the sub-chapter on the rings and diamond, I didn't know where to fit it in. This "Postscript" is sort of like an epilogue, so this section seems to be as good a place as any. And you can rest assured that I kept my promise to get my hand fixed. Tell me what you think when I finish reading it, honey. Here it goes.

Promises Kept

"For the last five or six years, my pinky, middle, and ring fingers of my left hand were curling, the tips toward my palm. My hand was partially disabled. The thumb and index fingers were not normally affected in cases of this disease, known as Dupuytren's contracture. If a person doesn't have it treated, the fingers can close tightly into the palm, and there may be no remedy. A surgeon would be unable to get the scalpel into a position to remove the diseased tissue that causes the problem.

"If the disease is not too far along, there is a needle procedure that sometimes works, thereby avoiding surgery. In my advanced condition, however, surgery was required. It was the constricting of the flexible tissue in the hand and fingers, not the tendons or the ligaments. The disease is extremely rare. It usually afflicts males a little later in life—fifties, sixties, or older. Its victims are most often of northern European descent, including Irish.

"It's also commonly known as Viking disease or Marauder's disease. So, somewhere in my ancestry, a battle-axe–toting, sword-swinging, probably fearsome warrior-oarsman, impregnated my g^{15}-mom as he swore oaths to Odin. You remember how my g-nieces referred to Pat and Don, their grandparents: "g-mom" and "g-pop." I probably cut the ancestry chain short. It may be to the two hundredth power, for all I know—maybe more.

"While Irene was ill, however, I needed both my hands. I couldn't have the surgery performed yet. Over that last five- or six-year period, we both watched my fingers curl a little more each year, often interfering with normal activities. It became something like a claw or a hook as the disease advanced. It doesn't hurt at all—not me, anyway. It is just very cumbersome."

Tom, I worried so much that you were waiting too long. I would have been fine for however long it took to get back to normal after surgery.

"I know. But I didn't want to take the risk of not being able to be of help to you."

Thank you, Tom.

"Okay. I'll continue now.

"I previously mentioned that Irene and I had our last pillow talk a few nights before she passed. She referenced the need for my surgery. She had me promise I would have it done after she passed. She wanted me to have my hand treated before it was too late. Instead of being a claw or hook, it would become a club. No wonder they call it Viking's disease.

"You may remember also that before Irene was diagnosed, we joked that she would take care of me in my old age. I was fifteen years older. She still tried to fulfill that mission, even while lying on her deathbed a few evenings before she died. She was still addressing my needs, not her own. Irene was always thinking of me, right to the very end.

"Well, in October 2012, I had the surgery. I kept my promise to Irene. At this writing, early 2013, I finished physical therapy, and my fingers are pointing straight up. I hadn't seen them in that position for a long time.

"Now, all I have to worry about regarding that disease is its return. It could happen.

"That's it, honey. That's the way I wrote it for your book."

I wish all of you could hear Irene—or can you? Her voice is so clear to me. Can you?

Good, Tom. I'm glad you kept that promise. You know, your hand always worried me. It seems like it will be fine.

"Yes, it will be, I know. But honey, I am so anxious for the swelling to go down, so I can wear our Claddagh on my left ring finger. It could be six months to a year, I'm told. I can't wear it on my right hand—it's too big. I don't want to lose it, you know. My left ring finger had that large disease-related knot in the segment where the ring fits. When it was first sized, it had to accommodate that lump. That accounted for the larger size. I miss wearing it, Irene. I might have to have it resized.

"So, all in all, hon, it's going well. I wear it a few hours each day, but then my finger starts to swell, so I take it off. It won't be long, though. I hope that fills you in enough, honey."

Thank you, handsome.

"I would like to add just a couple more little notes now, before I ask you several questions, sugar. There is something I really, really want to know, but it can wait. Please stay with me, Irene. Listen to this. It was something else I wrote but couldn't figure out where to include it in the book. This "Postscript" is coming in handy as an epilogue. Mike uses epilogues in his books, you know.

"I have acquired a habit I'm trying to break. You and I both had this habit, Irene. It's not serious. It just puts me out of sync with a large portion of the world. Here it goes.

Habits Acquired

"When Irene and I accepted the fact that she would be bedridden the majority of time, we bought the latest flat-screen, lightweight TVs for the family room and our bedroom. I wanted Irene to be comfortable. The lounge chair in the bedroom gave me the perch for reciting to her and for busying myself with my own interesting readings.

"However, as time passed and daylight waned, and then dusk and twilight filled our bedroom, I would muse over tangled thoughts of my own. Then, as darkness entered, I would lie down beside Irene. It felt like the right thing for me to do. I didn't want her to feel alone.

"We would watch the Cooking Channel through 8:00 PM and then channel surf until I found something intriguing, as Irene would close her eyes after meds and drift off into slumberland. Within an hour, after finishing anything that needed tending, I'd take my pills. My mind contemplated our situation and then, I'd drift off myself.

"That habit resulted in my being ready for the next day at 4:00 AM. Neither of us ever slept straight through. Sometimes, while Irene still slept, I waited for the doors to open at a busy family restaurant on 13th Street at 5:00 AM to have a quick breakfast. In the past, when Irene was ready for breakfast, I made it at home. Breakfast was the only meal I felt very confident in preparing."

Yes, Tom. You always made me tea and toast, too. Thank you.

"You're certainly welcome, my dear. Let me continue.

"Now that Irene has passed, I feel a general laziness or malaise. I go to that busy restaurant on 13th street for breakfast, instead of preparing it myself, and I am out the door before 5:00 AM. If I sometimes oversleep, I go to the restaurant on Pennsylvania Avenue that opens at 6:30 AM, where I chitchat with the owners. Then I return home and start writing.

"I'm now in the habit of spending a lot more money on breakfast and slipping into bed by 7:00 PM and watching TV. I can't bring myself to watch the Cooking Channel—it would bring back too many memories. In addition, I'm not capable of staying out once it gets dark, after not doing so for so long. Friends understand, and I am not ribbed for being an early-to-bed/early-to-rise individual, but it does commit me to limited exposure to the rest of the world—for now. I'm working on withholding my 5:00 PM yawns, delaying them for another hour or two—maybe when the book is completed."

That little piece is very quaint and cute, Tom. It's very short. It's not long at all, so you should include it in our book.

"Okay. Honey, I just wanted to comment on that sleeping thing. I got so used to falling asleep with the TV on that I still do that, too. As a matter of fact, I now need the TV on to get to sleep and to get back to sleep when I wake up in the middle of the night, just like you did. That habit is something I'm working on.

"But I have to tell you something else. We had a wonderful candlelight service at the funeral parlor a month ago. It was for all the souls who were laid to rest by that funeral home during 2012. A local pastor delivered a very compassionate sermon. The choir from St. Thomas Aquinas Church sang Christmas carols, and all during the ceremony, the photos of all the deceased individuals were shown on a widescreen TV. You looked terrific in your uniform photo, honey.

"Pat and Don were there. So were a couple friends of mine, Ed and Tim. Christmas season was difficult without you, honey. Your family invited me over there to Bradenton, but we were having a big get-together here. We all went to see *Les Misérables* at the Loop Mall on Christmas Day. Eleven of us occupied the last row, our favorite seats. There were a few very difficult scenes for me. Then we all went to the Orlando Ale House afterward for munchies.

The Calling

"But honey, now that I've brought you up-to-date, I have to know something. What were your thoughts? Not just at the final moments but those during the last few days. You were so weak that you were unable to speak to me. Did you know your sister was there at the end? Did you know I was holding your hand? Could you hear me saying that I love you? Was there anything I could have done for you?

"The end came so suddenly, honey. We thought we had at least another couple months to spend together, to talk of our past and of our love. I wasn't done caring for you. I wanted it to continue. Maybe you could have started eating that fish spread again—or cottage cheese. You did seem peaceful, except for those several last breaths.

"What did you see, honey? I could tell you were seeing something. Was it the bright light? I have a friend who saw it while he was comatose after an accident. You know, that bright light people talk about after having a near-death experience? They often become guests on the Oprah and Dr. Phil shows. I was asked about it after my surgery in 1990, when I was given the Last Rights of the Church. I never saw the light that everyone talks about. Maybe the light is different if you are sprawled on a highway, on an operating table, or in your own bed. Who knows? Did you see it, honey? Speak to me, Irene.

"Another thing that bothered me—I remember you often said you wanted a mass and a priest. You had the mass. Did you mean you wanted a priest to hear your last confession or to have the Last Rights? Were you afraid? We didn't have time to get a priest here. There was some confusion. But Irene, you were confessing for years to God, personally and directly! He heard you; I know. I've watched you devoutly praying for hours on end—your rosary, your novenas.

"Your soul was pure when you left this life, honey. You needn't have been afraid. My brother would tell us that it is an imperfect contrition if we confess out of fear. Your conversations with God were well-received, I'm sure. You were praying out of love, too, not fear. You told me so. Who could not have loved you? You taught everyone whose life you touched how to love. Your constant concern for me and Maria made me understand, in my old age, what real true love can be: unselfish, generous, giving, and comforting. No one could love as deeply as you loved. We all miss you so much.

"Please speak to me, honey. Don't go yet. Please.

"When you came into my life I was in a situation absent of the love of a woman. I didn't think there could be a woman for me to love, so I reconciled myself to a life of work and dedication to my sons. When you entered my world, I was reborn. It happened without fanfare, and it was so natural when I realized I was in love with you. You were a keeper. I had no doubt.

"Please, honey, speak to me of your thoughts. How were you viewing the world around you? I remember how you smiled whenever we toured and wherever we went. You grasped every sunrise and sunset as though it was your last. I realize now you were preparing to die and wanted to leave life with positive and beautiful feelings about the world around you. Everyone could learn from you, honey. Teach them now—through your book. Tell them how to live. Show them how to fight. Teach them how to die, Irene. Please.

"Your smile was so natural, it would be out of character for you to be gloomy toward the end of your life. Are you happy? Will I be with you once more, forever? Please speak to me."

Yes, Tom. I heard your loving words as you held my hand. I am happy now and without pain.

The light protects. It absorbs pain. It is heavenly. It is beatific. Those breaths you heard were my body breathing its last, Tom, not my soul. In my case, my soul was protected by the light. To others it may mean something else. To me, it was peaceful and protective. It's the natural process of dying.

You gave me the most precious and expensive gift any human being can give to another. You gave of your time, Tom, your time—the most expensive and most appreciated gift of all. The gift of time! That was your time that you unselfishly gave in the waning years of your own life. You fulfilled my life, knowing that I was loved so deeply. Tom, I hear them calling.

"Who, honey? Who is calling? Don't leave me yet, honey. Irene?"

Yes, Tom. I'm here. But I'm not sure for how long. Please, Tom. I loved when you would read to me, and I still do. Please, will you recite my favorite Shakespeare, if you have re-remembered the sonnet? Remember that time when you told me you would recite it to me after you re-remembered it? That was so endearing, Tom. Will you?

"I sure will, honey. That sonnet exactly described how I felt when I knew I was in love with you. The poet says he longed to have gifts that others had, like art and physical features. He was very down on himself too. He didn't think he had any value in the eyes of the world. His cries to heaven for a better life went unheard. He couldn't feel content with anything. In other words, like me at the time, there wasn't a woman for him to love in his world. But then, someone came into his life."

Please hurry, handsome. I hear something going on in the distance.

"Okay, listen, honey. I mean every word of this sonnet. Before I met you, I was so emotionally starved that I thought I would never find the love of a woman again."

Hurry, Tom. Hurry, please!

> "When in disgrace with fortune and men's eyes,
> I all alone beweep my outcast state
> And trouble deaf heaven with my bootless cries
> And look upon myself and curse my fate,
> Wishing me like to one more rich in hope,
> Featured like him, like him with friends possess'd,
> Desiring this man's art and that man's scope,
> With what I most enjoy contented least;
> Yet in these thoughts myself almost despising,
> Haply I think on thee, and then my state,
> Like to the lark at break of day arising
> From sullen earth, sings hymns at heaven's gate;
> For thy sweet love remember'd such wealth brings
> That then I scorn to change my state with kings."

That was beautiful, as always. You must have re-remembered it. I love you so much, Tom, and I always will. Thank you for that. I'll always treasure the love you had for me. We entered each other's lives at the very best moment for each of us. Tom! Tom! I hear them calling.

"Please, honey. Not yet. I need more answers. I need more answers."

I hear them calling. I think I hear them calling me, Tom. Do you hear them?

"No!"

Yes! I hear them calling me! Me! We will be together again. Now I'm certain of it, Tom. I will see you again, darling. I love you! Whoopee!

Honey … sugar … beautiful … Irene? Irene?

⚜

More Reviews and Comments…

"… I just finished it a few days ago…Once I started reading it I knew I had to finish it… I think you really captured how much you and Irene loved each other…She was so brave…You really let everyone in on your private life… I know that must have been hard…." --F.D.

"For anyone who believes in love you must read this book. Irene was the sweetest person and Tom is great person who loved Irene. Their struggle was hard but love and family got them through the tough times." --MB.C.

"…Soul Mates, a mystery, or makes you smile and kiss your partner? ... Surely, cancer has touched your Life in one form or another. If you, your significant other, a family member, neighbor, friend - or if you want to learn the depths of what the battle can be - you must read this book." -J.C.

"Just finished reading Tom Cooney's new book. I recommend it to anyone who has been truly in love (soul mate), or has had a battle with cancer. It would be very helpful to caregivers. priceless information." --M.C.

"…A stunning book introducing Irene Cooney through the eyes of her adoring husband; he was hooked by her winning smile and fell into a love for all time! A must read for all who love a true love story. A "should read" for anyone wanting a roadmap to the courage and selflessness it takes to do what Tom Cooney has done!" --P.L.

"Love shows no boundaries in this beautiful story of a 4th stage cancer patient who would endure years of hospital stays, countless operations, over 175 chemo treatments, swallowed thousands of pills and always had the attitude "I want quantity of life…" --D. & P.McG.

"Tom, your book is the best book I ever read... I feel as though I know her very well. The two of you had something very precious. At times my wife asked if I was ok because she could see I was being affected...I laughed, too. At times the humor came through--at the right times." --L.L.

"Tom, the book was great. You and Irene really had something special. I was so moved by it. My wife wants to read it too." --J.F.

"Tom, Irene and you were a beautiful couple. I know she's a good listener and has a lot of influence now ... so I'm talking!!!!" --Love ya Moe.

"Hi Tom. I finished the book!!!! I loved it as much as I love Irene! ... I cried most of the time, ... I will reread it soon ..." --Love N.D.

"A moving true-love story of loyalty, commitment and hope." –Anon.

And many more....

Visit the Website:

http://www.CancerA9YearStruggle.com

Listen to Irene and Tom's favorite love ballads as soon as you open it. It contains much behind the scenes information that can be used to enhance your experience of reading the book. The website contains several pages: Home, About the Book, Inside the Book, Photos (more than 100 pictures), Comments and Reviews, About the Author, and a Contact page to send Tom your thoughts.

Made in United States
Troutdale, OR
11/03/2026

56844358R00177